Using Spirituality in Psychotherapy

Using Spirituality in Psychotherapy: The Heart Led Approach to Clinical Practice offers a means for therapists to integrate a spiritual perspective into their clinical practice.

The book provides a valuable alternative to traditional forms of psychotherapy by placing an emphasis on purpose and meaning. Introducing a spiritually informed model, Heart Led Psychotherapy (HLP), the book uses a BioPsychoSocioSpiritual approach to treat psychological distress. Based on the premise that everyone is on an individual life journey, HLP teaches clients to become an observer, identifying the life lessons that they are being asked to understand or experience. The model can be used whether a client has spiritual beliefs or not, enabling them to make new choices that are in keeping with their authentic selves and to live a more fulfilled and peaceful life. This new edition includes updated references and new material on transpersonal psychology, spiritual awakening, working within the quantum field, significance of the heart and heart coherence.

Illustrated by case studies to highlight key points and including a range of practical resource exercises and strategies, this engaging book will have wide appeal to ` therapists and clinicians from a variety of backgrounds.

Dr Alexandra Dent is a Registered and Chartered Clinical Psychologist working with individuals across the age span in Independent Practice in the East Midlands, UK. Areas of interest include trauma, attachment, mindfulness, and spirituality. Alexandra is an active member of the EMDR community and is a Europe Accredited EMDR Child and Adolescent Consultant, EMDR Consultant and Training Facilitator, and Chair of the Special Interest Group in EMDR & Spirituality.

'An insightful and valuable contribution to the emerging field of spiritually informed psychotherapy.'

Philip Carr-Gomm, *psychologist and psychosynthesis psychotherapist*

'This book is authentic, inspiring and beautifully written. The book clearly demonstrates how HLP works in practice and can be combined with other therapies including mindfulness. The author reveals her own spiritual journey with courage and truth and encourages readers to explore their own spirituality, opening an important doorway for further exploration of their own Self. The book is full of "heart".'

Michelle Sorrell, *author of* The Wonder of Stillness, Meditation for Children, A Practical Guide for Parents and Teachers

Praise for the first edition

'This is an excellent book introducing a new spiritually informed Heart Led Psychotherapy which integrates solid trauma healing with a spiritual based perspective of soul awareness and life lessons. Alexandra Dent explains the evolving role of the therapist as a guide into the deeper wounds of the heart and soul with a clear step-by-step protocol which is used as part of a BioPsychoSocialSpiritual model to understand life challenges and traumas. In particular, she illustrates how Heart Led Psychotherapy can be used in conjunction with EMDR, enabling multi-dimensional healing. A must read for therapists and clients alike interested in the expanding context of psychotherapy.'

Irene R. Siegel, Ph.D., LCSW; *approved EMDR consultant; author of* The Sacred Path of the Therapist: Modern Healing, Ancient Wisdom, and Client Transformation

'Heart Led Psychotherapy (HLP) helps clients go beyond the limitations of their ego into the greener pastures of their heart and soul. This model recognises a broader perspective of life in that life is always presenting opportunities and challenges to help us connect more deeply to our authentic core. Life will inevitably present lessons that are there to help us grow. All challenging experiences, relationships, or traumas are opportunities to experience these lessons. Also, choices made from the heart lead to better outcomes than choices made from the head or ego. Sometimes such choices will require a releasing of the old and a leap of faith into the new. Making such a choice will always lead to a more authentic life. Alexandra's inclusion of the spiritual dimension in the HLP model is probably a much welcome breath of fresh air for any therapist wishing to include the spiritual dimension in their therapeutic work.'

Steve Nobel, *author, spiritual coach and creator of* The Soul Matrix healing system

Using Spirituality in Psychotherapy

The Heart Led Approach to Clinical Practice

Second Edition

Alexandra Dent

Routledge
Taylor & Francis Group

LONDON AND NEW YORK

Designed cover image: Getty Images

Second edition published 2026
by Routledge
4 Park Square, Milton Park, Abingdon, Oxon, OX14 4RN

and by Routledge
605 Third Avenue, New York, NY 10158

Routledge is an imprint of the Taylor & Francis Group, an informa business

First edition published by Routledge 2020

British Library Cataloguing-in-Publication Data
A catalogue record for this book is available from the British Library

ISBN: 978-1-041-01222-1 (hbk)
ISBN: 978-1-041-01221-4 (pbk)
ISBN: 978-1-003-61374-9 (ebk)

DOI: 10.4324/9781003613749

Typeset in Times New Roman
by codeMantra

Access the Support Material: www.routledge.com/9781041012214

To my beautiful children, Olivia and Sebastian.

Contents

Figures and table

Figures

Table

Foreword

Alexandra has introduced therapists to the important concept of incorporating a spiritual dimension into their work with clients, having developed a new spiritually informed psychotherapy, Heart Led Psychotherapy (HLP). Within this, two working models are presented: a Heart Led (HL) or Heart and Soul Led (HASL) model. This sees spirituality as all-embracing and inclusive of all beliefs and in those with none. At the most basic level it is related to the Latin *spiritus* meaning to breathe. The ancient Sanskrit word *Dharma* is defined as, 'an inner calling that your heart knows.' Thus, the wisdom of the heart acts as a counterbalance to the rationalism of the left hemisphere dominated Western civilisation. The *soul* is defined as 'an immortal, invisible energy, the Divine within us that originated from the Divine Source of unconditional love.' Our soul is contained in a physical body. A path toward exploration of spirituality is outlined. This can lead to the development of intuition, which is often felt at the level of the third eye chakra. The HL approach can be extended to the HASL model, which incorporates an exploration of the role of soul in the client's life.

A BioPsychoSocioSpiritual approach to treating psychological distress is explained as part of HLP. This can be incorporated with other therapies such as Eye Movement Desensitisation and Reprocessing (EMDR). With EMDR, a transpersonal psychology approach is combined with spiritual interweaves. These involve listening to your heart and soul, understanding life lessons and the relevance of this experience for healing, learning, and making meaning. Each client can be introduced to a spiritually informed approach to therapy in the early stages of their therapeutic path. This can lay the foundation for post traumatic growth and optimal performance in the future.

The role of the ego is analysed and its expectations can be overcome in the sense that egocentricities are dispensed with and the heartfelt connections are initiated and projected outwards going forward. Letting go of the ego opens up the path to heartfelt conversations and therapist and client connect 'heart to heart.' The ultimate aim of HLP is helping clients live a more authentic life time.

Mindfulness has a key role to play in HLP. It creates an enhanced state of conscious awareness and acts as a buffer against traumatic dissociation. This book introduces narratives for the client, which help to activate this state during the therapeutic process. The meditative aspects include: awareness, acceptance, compassion, being non-judgemental, with a script for mindful breathing. These exercises are explained so that therapists with little experience of these ideas can easily build them into their clinical practice. Finally, it is essential for therapists to practice what they preach so that they have an embodied sense of purpose in the clinical setting.

This book delves into the research on the benefits of living with a concept of your heart and soul. Wilber in 2000 and Father Paul Hyland have written about the whispers of my soul. This I believe shows the connectedness of all human existence both past, present and in the future at the level of quantum consciousness. Various strategies and exercises are described enabling the reader to become more aware of the influence of heart and soul mindfulness on their current life issues. The concept of enriching and draining aspects of the client's life is visualised. Each client's experience of embracing a spiritual aspect to the therapeutic consultation is an individual one in the first instance. While initially seeking happiness as an outcome, it is likely that they emerge in a state of grace, self-love, and tranquillity. The soul becomes aligned with the Divine Source and can exist in a state of bliss, freedom, and authenticity. This is similar to the *wu wei* concept of non-action, non-doing, and non-forcing described by Lao Tzu in Taoism. People who wish to embrace a heart and soul based life often have to take a leap of faith. Although challenging the case histories described throughout this book prove it to be a rewarding experience.

The different stages of the HL and HASL models are described in detail. This involves identifying challenges faced by the client at several levels. These are moved from a cognitive frame of reference to a heart and soul based one. Fundamental to this transition is becoming the observer, not the observed. This has similarities to the basic rest activity cycle described by Professor Ernest Rossi. The life lessons learned along the way help this process to become established at a heart and soul level. The key to successful post traumatic growth is to turn these life lessons into gifts of insight and awareness.

One of the innovations of this book is the detailed explanation of HLP so that clients can inform themselves of the stages of the process. This is on the basis of a script, which can lead to a more authentic life. Clients are encouraged to become the observer, identify the life lessons and explore the gifts that have led to greater authenticity. The end result should be greater intuition and insight.

The book includes a discussion on the origin of souls and how souls can work together as a family to teach, learn and heal. It is believed that certain therapists who work with soul energy and cosmic vibrations are themselves connected at a soul level. The idea of soul level blocks and restrictions are explained. This brings up the diverse issues of trauma at a soul level and what is recorded and accessible in the Akashic Records. If clients are interested guidance is given on how to pursue these areas further. Advanced techniques include: shamanic healing, soul retrieval, past life regression, soul readings, and karmic influences.

Alexandra takes the brave step in her book of articulating her own spiritual journey as evidence of how she walked the walk. I think as therapists we should all be prepared to articulate our own vulnerabilities. This shows clients the journey involved in our own path toward living an authentic life.

For Carl Jung,

> a good half of every treatment that probes at all deeply consists in the doctor's examining himself … it is his own hurt that gives a measure of his power to heal.
>
> (Jung quoted in Anthony Stevens, *Jung*, Oxford, 1994, p. 110)

In summary, this book is essential reading for all therapists wishing to embrace a spiritual dimension into their therapeutic work with clients.

Art O'Malley, author of *Sensorimotor-Focused EMDR: A New Paradigm for Psychotherapy and Peak Performance* (2018)

Preface

It's your road and yours alone. Others may walk it with you, but no one can walk it for you.

Rumi

Hello heart.

As of now I am making peace with my heart centre, I must be able to forgive those who have abused my heart. My heart is not deserving of this. My heart is my truth, but I am forgiving you my heart because I feel here you have led me astray. I want you to know heart centre, that I am just so angry. I feel so beaten. I feel so exposed. I feel so raw. But now I work with you heart centre to find my truth and I am going to stop blaming you for leading me astray because I feel that you have lied to me and I have felt so out of alignment with you, my beating heart and my beating soul, and I now need to forgive myself of this judgement and this cross I bear. I am aware now that my heart centre does not lie to me, that my heart centre guides me, and that my heart heals and that my heart will always see me right, but I have just struggled to be able to see that. Now I see that and I welcome you back in heart centre, because for years I have felt angry toward you and I have felt as though you have been outside of my body, but what I now understand is that you will not see me wrong. I salute and embrace you because you give me the life force to create and understand that my life is magical and it doesn't matter where other people's heart centres are. It is not my responsibility and I must not take responsibility for fixing their hearts and their wounds. I see now heart centre where my problem has lain. I have put you in a box. I have labelled you and for that I am truly sorry. I now work with your magical vibrancy to burst forward with joy, creativity and expression and I thank you for this time as I talk to you today.

The above transcript came from an angelic reiki healing session I had while writing this book.

'You had to walk the walk to talk the talk.' This was the message I was given by several spiritual mentors over the years. I had to go through my own personal challenges as well as developing a clinical way of working with clients that incorporated spirituality in order to develop a new model of working so that I could share my experiences with a wider audience and demonstrate some credibility behind my message.

Toward the end of 2017 and the beginning of 2018, I was also told by four separate spiritual advisors that there was a book within me that was long overdue. I know that being concise and articulate is not my *forté* and I would never pride myself on being very eloquent with words, so to write a book seemed like a daunting and unachievable task. It still took some time before a light bulb turned on and I realised that if the universe wanted me to write a book and share my spiritual work in a purely academic way, they would have given me these abilities to begin with! So perhaps this book was meant to be written simply, so that the message can be easily understood and be available to everyone, without being complicated by fancy jargon. I was also meant to learn self-belief during this process and not judge myself or worry about the judgements others may have if they were dissatisfied or disagreed with the content of the book; I had to learn to let go of judgement and just trust.

What I hadn't quite established was the content of the book. I knew my clinical psychology work mostly focused on trauma and attachment issues, especially utilising mindfulness, attachment work, and Eye Movement Desensitisation and Reprocessing (EMDR) in the therapy I delivered. However, my real passion and drive went beyond this, because I wanted to get an understanding of individuals' life stories from a more holistic and spiritual perspective. There just seemed to be a missing part of the jigsaw puzzle when formulating clinical presentations using a traditional approach. So often in the Western psychotherapeutic world we just don't ask any questions about people's spiritual beliefs or consciously work at a heart and soul level and yet this can have a considerable influence on how individuals view themselves, their situations, and their experiences and become a very powerful and positive resource. It is as if there is an underlying *fear* that asking such questions will open up a can of worms that no one will know how to deal with.

For many years I have been acutely aware of a change in the type of individuals attending my clinics. I never used to advertise or refer to my spirituality or how I worked in this way, yet the more open I became about introducing this concept into my work the more I found that clients who were ready to explore a spiritual angle to their difficulties were finding their way to my clinics. I have also heard of clients who actively seek therapists who incorporate spirituality into sessions, as this can be such a significant and empowering part of their healing.

In 2016, I was introduced to healing at a soul level. I felt a huge awakening and understanding of what my soul journey was about and I felt I started to gain a greater understanding of all of the challenges that I had experienced in this lifetime, including relationships and situations that I had found myself in. I soon observed a mirroring with the knowledge and healing I was gaining through my own spiritual discovery and the difficulties my clients were experiencing. The more comfortable I became about introducing spirituality into sessions, the more clients also seemed more open and interested in this approach, many of whom became curious about additional healing at a soul level. This has been a wonderful and enriching experience because I witnessed clients heal at a multi-dimensional level.

This book has been part of my spiritual journey; introducing Heart Led Psychotherapy (HLP), a spiritually informed psychotherapy, which provides a pathway to helping individuals live an authentic life through their heart and soul. Part 1 discusses how to introduce spirituality into your clinical work and introduces a BioPsychoSocioSpiritual approach to treating psychological distress. Part 2 then focuses on the role of the ego in psychological distress and teaches clients how to move away from their ego and learn how to live a mindful life from their heart and soul. Part 3 describes fully the process of HLP and how to implement HLP with your clients. It concludes with a chapter on who may benefit from HLP, possible awakening symptoms that may occur when someone embarks on a spiritual journey, tips to look after yourself as a therapist and how to apply HLP in supervision. Part 4 provides three detailed case illustrations of HLP, a supervision case and a summary of my own personal journey. All the additional resources required can be found in Part 5. Case examples are used throughout the book to illustrate certain areas. Client's names have been anonymised to respect their privacy, but all have given permission for their stories to be shared.

At this point I think it is important to emphasise that spirituality is a very personal area and there are many different ideas, concepts and beliefs that exist in the world. My spiritual beliefs, which have developed through my own journey and discoveries, resonate with me but I have had to go through my own process of exploration and experimentation to eliminate areas that I don't feel comfortable with and expand on areas that I connect with more strongly. Even since the first edition of this book, some of my beliefs have changed and I feel that this update represents a much more authentic version of myself. I am still learning and there is so much more for me to discover and understand. Therefore, it is essential that if interested in this area, each person finds what resonates with them. The underpinnings of HLP are spiritually informed and based on some of the spiritual concepts I have discovered so far. It is not the intention of this book to suggest that these spiritual concepts are facts or the ultimate truth and that would also be impossible to prove! However, the spiritual concepts I have drawn upon have provided the framework for HLP which aims to support clients to find and then deepen their self-love and live an authentic life in whatever capacity that may be. For those who believe in the presence of a soul, then HLP can also guide clients to live a heart and soul led life, again developing self-love and their own authenticity.

It is beyond the remit of this book to provide a detailed review of any historical, philosophical, spiritual, religious, and mystical teachings, but for anyone who is interested, there is a wealth of information available elsewhere. This is also not an academic book full of intellectual jargon or references but instead provides a working model with the information and resources required to use HLP with clients if you so choose. It is written from my heart and soul based on my own personal, clinical and spiritual journey throughout this time. I hope that I will be able to deliver a simple message that is easy to understand and accessible to all. Some key messages are repeated throughout the book; this is intentional, as I want to really highlight the significance of these points in HLP.

Acknowledgements

First, I want to thank all the clients that I have ever worked with. It has been such an honour and privilege and is always a humbling experience when clients can find trust in me and open up to reveal their struggles and vulnerability. I hope that I never take this for granted, but always appreciate the beautiful gift you give back to me in this process. An especially big thank you to those clients who agreed to be case studies for this book. My writing continued to evolve as our sessions progressed. The enthusiasm you have shown for Heart Led Psychology and your active involvement and commitment has been so touching.

Second, a special thank you goes to the amazing healers who have supported me on my spiritual journey, who have been my lifesavers at times. Especially Liz King, my spiritual guide, friend and colleague; you have been my rock. You have been there for me far beyond what I could ever imagine, through some very dark places. I will never forget your kindness and support and I simply love working with you – you are a great inspiration and have also helped so many of my clients with their journeys too. A huge thank you to Patsy Shillinglaw and Ralph Ticehurst for their wonderful guidance and healing over the past few years and for keeping me afloat and believing in me. I would also like to thank Dr Harmony, who I have only known a short while, but connecting with you and embarking on your 12 session 'Reboot Your Soul' programme enabled me to complete some essential healing and gain deeper understanding and facilitated this book to start taking shape and form.

A massive thank you must be extended to Irene Siegel. You have been such a supportive and encouraging influence over the past few years and took time out of your busy schedule to read the book and provide fantastic constructive feedback. I am truly grateful. A big thank you also extends to Art O'Malley who kindly agreed to write a foreword for this book.

I would like to say a special thanks to my colleagues and friends on the UK EMDR Child & Adolescent Committee between 2016 and 2021. During my time on this committee, we all worked exceptionally hard on a voluntary basis because we believed in the powerful healing of EMDR. I am so proud to have known you all, you have such gentle souls and it was a pleasure to work alongside you and for such a great cause. While we were determined to work hard, we also managed to hold a lightness and sense of fun and humour.

I have some very close special friends who have also been there for me at key points on my journey. It would be too difficult to mention all your names and I fear I may miss someone out and wound their hearts. You know who you are! I feel truly blessed to have you in my life.

To one of my dear friends, Nicki Fayers, who helped me edit the first edition. We laughed together at my Dyslexic phrases and spellings and you have provided great wisdom and insight. Your support with the book came at just the right time and in answer to my request to the universe for help! I cherish you as the loving, wonderful friend that you are and also admire your strength, courage, and bravery to live your life through your heart too.

To my gorgeous, adorable children, Olivia and Sebastian. When you were born you brought a healing of its own kind. I recognised you both when I first laid eyes on you – we have had many past lives together. You are my treasures, I am so proud of you both, for the strength and determination and spark that you shine out to the world. I love you both equally. May you always find a way of living through your heart and soul and may you be blessed with love, grace and peace.

Finally, I would like to thank all the universal support that has been available to me throughout my life, especially while writing this book. This includes but is not limited to my own personal team of guides, teachers, angels, and archangels. I believe that I have just been a vessel or channel for the content of this book but the actual wisdom has come from the Divine Source.

Part 1

Introducing a spiritual perspective into psychotherapy

1

Spiritual work with clients

Be drunk with love, for love is all that exists.

Rumi

This chapter discusses a transpersonal approach within psychotherapy and explores some of the different meanings of spirituality and the soul. Guidance is then provided on how you can explore your own beliefs about spirituality before introducing these ideas to your clients. The benefits of working spiritually with clients are discussed, which also includes accessing additional, positive spiritual resources. Heart Led Psychotherapy (HLP) is introduced as a new spiritually informed therapy that has two working models: the first is a Heart Led (HL) model that can be used with any client regardless of their spiritual beliefs, and the second is a Heart and Soul Led (HASL) model that can be applied to those clients open to the concept of a soul. The key spiritual concepts for both models are also detailed, which include the idea that life is an individual journey in which challenges, traumas, and attachment/relationship difficulties can provide opportunities to understand and experience life lessons in order to find self-love and live a more authentic life that is in keeping with the heart and soul.

Transpersonal psychology

Transpersonal psychology evolved in the 1960s and 1970s as a branch within psychology that adopted a spiritual, transcendent, and transformational way to understand and explore human experiences and psychological distress. It is now considered the Fourth Force in Psychology, where psychology has moved from a behavioural to a psychoanalytical, to a humanistic, and finally a transpersonal approach. Walsh and Vaughan (1993, p. 203) defined transpersonal psychology as:

> experiences in which the sense of identity or self extends beyond (trans) the individual or personal to encompass wider aspects of humankind, life, psyche or cosmos.

DOI: 10.4324/9781003613749-2

Caplan (2009, p. 231) suggested:

> Transpersonal psychologists attempt to integrate timeless wisdom and mod-
> ern Western psychology and translate spiritual principles into scientifically
> grounded, contemporary language. Transpersonal psychology addresses the full
> spectrum of human psychospiritual development – from our deepest wounds
> and needs, to the existential crisis of human being, to the most transcendent
> capacities of our consciousness.

Transpersonal psychology aims to integrate the more traditional psychological approaches with spiritual and mystical experiences, including religious and philosophical traditions. It bridges together Eastern and Western practices and ideas,
science and spirituality to cultivate personal and collective transformation. It also
attempts to move away from a dualistic perspective towards nondualism in the pur-
suit of self-actualisation or enlightenment by exploring experiences that transcend
the ego or self-identity.

One of the earliest contributors to the foundation of transpersonal psychology,
dating back to the 19th century, was William James. A philosopher and psychologist, James is considered by many to be the founder of American psychology,
encouraging an open and pragmatic approach to philosophy and incorporating
subjective experiences of individuals in religious or mystical states into his work.
Another significant key contributor to the transpersonal psychology movement was
Carl Jung in the 20th century. Jung is famous for his work on the concepts of
collective consciousness and archetypes which evolved through his own personal
spiritual journey, dream analysis, as well as spiritual training with Indian Hindu
gurus. The term 'collective unconscious' is a concept introduced by Jung (1959a)
to describe the part of the unconscious mind that universally connects individuals
to a shared human psyche inherent in all cultures, history and archetypes rather
than acquired through personal experiences. An archetype represents a universal
symbol, pattern, or theme that appears across culture and throughout history which
can shape human experiences and may emerge in dreams, myths, art, or religion.
Archetypes are considered both permanent and evolving, help to give meaning to
the world, and can trigger a deep unconscious response in a person. They can hold
a numinous quality that may be Divine, spiritual, or religious, sometimes moving
beyond ordinary states of comprehension, activating powerful emotions and experiences. Archetypal crises may occur when numinous experiences are felt but then
not integrated fully into present-day life.

Jung's four main archetypes are the Self, Shadow, Persona, and Anima/Animus,
but other familiar ones include the Hero, People Pleaser, Mother, Rescuer, and
Trickster. The 'Self' represents the integration and unity of the unconscious and
conscious to bring about wholeness. While Jung believed that the Self transcends
the ego (or conscious identity), he also included it as one of the Self's components.
He felt that when the ego was in dialogue with the Self, this facilitated individuals to
align their conscious values to a deeper wisdom of the unconscious, enabling them

to connect with their own unique identity, enhance self-awareness, wholeness and balance in life, a process he described as 'individuation.' Jung used the 'Shadow' archetype to describe the darker side of the Self, the part that isn't liked, is hidden away, or avoided both within oneself and from the outside world. Jung believed that an essential part of the spiritual journey required practising self-awareness, connecting and integrating the Shadow, and aligning with the Self to enable one to live a more authentic life.

One pivotal individual who was influenced by Jung's work and who made a substantial contribution to the transpersonal evolution was Joseph Campbell. Campbell was a world-famous writer and mythologist and probably best known for his work the 'Hero's Journey' (which can be found in his volume *The Hero with a Thousand Faces*, Campbell, 2012). In this narrative, he described how a protagonist went on an adventure and faced various challenges and experiences that mirrored the universal human journey of struggle. During this journey, the protagonist gained insights, growth, and transformation by overcoming adversity. This powerful narrative resonates with many individuals on a spiritual journey as it highlights the necessity of moving away from a sense of comfort and familiarity to venture into the unknown. By increasing one's self-awareness, opportunities to experience and learn important life lessons are created. When this learning is integrated, transformation is possible.

Other early key contributors to the transpersonal psychology movement include:

1. Roberto Assagioli, an Italian psychiatrist and psychoanalyst who recognised the significance of the higher self and spiritual development within therapy. Integrating spiritual concepts within a psychotherapeutic framework, he developed Psychosynthesis in the early 20th century which particularly focused on personal growth, self-awareness and the integration of all aspects of an individual as a whole; body, emotions, mind and spirit.
2. Abraham Maslow, an American psychologist, best known for co-founding the Humanistic Psychology movement and introducing the concept of self-actualisation to describe the process in which an individual can reach their true full potential.
3. Stanislav Grof, an American psychiatrist, whose research in the use of psychedelics, in particular lysergic acid diethylamide (LSD), demonstrated how individuals experienced profound spiritual and transpersonal states. He also explored the benefits of psychedelic-assisted psychotherapy to treat various mental health conditions. Grof went on to develop Holotropic Breathwork, a technique that enables individuals to access non-ordinary states of consciousness without the need to use psychedelics.
4. Ken Wilber, a contemporary American psychologist and philosopher, known for blending Eastern spiritual traditions with Western psychology to create his famous Integral Model. This model provides a comprehensive holistic framework to understand human development and experience and has a broader application than Psychosynthesis, being applicable to areas such as education, business and much more.

The process of spiritual awakening

The famous Sufi mystic and poet Rumi, and the Indian spiritual master Sathya Sai Baba described three main stages during the awakening process:

1. Awareness to presence outside of oneself.
2. Awareness to presence within oneself.
3. 'I am' presence, in other words nondual awareness.

Using an example of learning to connect with the Divine Source, initially a person will recognise the Divine Source as outside of themselves, then move into acknowledging the Divine within themselves. Lastly, they are able to transcend the world they reside in; they are the Divine.

The spiritual awakening process can be very personal and transformative and experienced in various different ways. It involves transcending the ego to connect with a deeper sense of purpose, self, and the universe. Steve Taylor (2017) described the spiritual journey as a form of awakening. In order to stay awake, one has to first leave a state of sleep, metaphorically keep eyes open and stay connected to the present moment. In some individuals the spiritual awakening process may manifest suddenly, often as a result of a significant life event or spiritual experience that causes a profound shift in consciousness or awareness. Psychological distress and trauma have been shown to be some of the key triggers to a spontaneous spiritual awakening, enabling an individual to go within themselves in order to find meaning from such challenges (Taylor & Egeto-Szabo, 2017; Taylor, 2019). For others, the process may be gentler and over a longer period of time as various gained insights or changes in perspective become integrated within the Self.

Some recognised different forms of spiritual awakening include:

- Near Death Experience (NDE).
- Dark Night of the Soul: a challenging period of time where beliefs, attachments, and identity are challenged, often involving suffering and a sense of confusion and isolation.
- Kundalini awakening, where the Kundalini energy, believed by mystical and yogi traditions to reside at the base of the spine, becomes activated and moves up the energy centres (chakras) in the spine, resulting in an increase in awareness, consciousness and connection with the cosmos.
- Spiritual crisis or emergency: a term introduced by Grof and Grof (2010) to explain a sudden and intense identity crisis, often as a result of a spiritual experience, where one's meaning system drastically alters and may disrupt an individual's cognitive, emotional, and physical functioning.

White (1994) coined the term 'Exceptional Human Experiences' (EHE) to account for different reported extraordinary experiences reported by individuals that transcend ordinary understanding and perceptions, creating a lasting impression on an individual's life. Examples include telepathy, clairvoyance, synchronicity, precognition, psychokinesis, NDEs, out-of-body experiences, altered states of consciousness, Kundalini awakening, mystical experiences, and encounters with apparitions or ghosts. Grof and Grof (2010) suggested that there are two distinct ways in which spiritual experiences can occur. They termed the first way as the 'immanent Divine' where an individual views themselves as part of a unified field of cosmic creative energy; they are at one with everything around them. Everything is understood as an expression of themselves and any perceived boundaries are viewed as unreal or an illusion. The second way, the 'transcendental Divine,' is where an individual transcends linear time, the everyday world and state of consciousness in order to connect with archetypal beings, different realms, ancestors, the collective unconscious, racial and karmic patterns and phylogenetic sequences.

The quantum field

David Bohm (1917–1992) is recognised as a key physicist and philosopher whose work in quantum theory, consciousness and philosophy made significant contributions and insights into our understanding of quantum mechanics and quantum theory. He explored fundamental questions about the nature of reality, consciousness, and human experience, viewing the universe as a complex, infinite, multidimensional, multi-layered thought form. Some of his groundbreaking ideas include the notion of an implicate order and holomovement. The implicate order proposes that there is a hidden order containing the potential for all things, where everything is interconnected and from where deeper underlying reality emerges. The explicate order arises from the implicate order and is the reality we perceive in which everyday experiences are manifested. Bohm used the term 'holomovement' to describe the process by which the implicate and explicate orders interact, suggesting that the universe is in a constant state of flux and interconnectedness, where every part of existence dynamically relates to every other part, transcending space and time.

Laszlo (2009) introduced the term '*biofield*' to describe a subtle universal energy field that surrounds and impregnates all living organisms. This biofield unites energy and consciousness, connecting all living systems to a larger universe that extends beyond the body, environment, time, and space. Dispenza (2017) has become renowned for his work on the mind–body connection and the transformative potential of the quantum field, combining ideas from quantum physics, neuroplasticity, epigenetics and heart–brain coherence. He suggests the quantum field exists in the 5th dimension and is beyond time, space and ego, whereas individuals in physical form currently reside in the 3rd dimension (3D). The quantum field cannot be experienced through our senses; it is only blackness and is sometimes referred to as the 'zero point' field. One can only enter the quantum field through awareness or consciousness by releasing all connection and attachment to the physical 3D world, moving from a place of being 'somebody' to 'nobody.' Dispenza advocates that within the quantum field all possibilities, knowledge, dimensions, realms, space, energy and frequency exist and by entering and interacting with this quantum field, one can consciously change their reality. He provides ideas and techniques to assist this process which include mindfulness and meditation, visualisation and intention, enhancing one's emotional energy and reconditioning the mind and body.

What is spirituality?

You may be wondering why it is necessary or desirable to work using a spiritual or transpersonal approach. From my own personal experience, as well as working with clients, I have come to realise and appreciate that incorporating spirituality into clinical work not only accesses and utilises positive resources for an individual, but it can potentially facilitate a transformative process that allows the possibility of healing at a multi-dimensional level. Spirituality has been acknowledged by The World Health Organization as an important factor of mental health since 1984 at their 37th Assembly and on quality of life in 2006 (The WHOQOL SRPB Group, 2006). In 1994, the category of 'Religious or Spiritual Problem' was introduced into the *Diagnostic and Statistical Manual of Mental Disorders-4* (DSM-4) referring to religious or spiritual problems as non-pathological problems that resulted in distress, such as loss of faith, converting to a new faith, or questioning of spiritual values (American Psychiatric Association, 1994). In 2013, the Royal College of Psychiatrists produced recommendations for psychiatrists on spirituality and religion. The formation of specialist interest groups and committees for clinicians in the area of spirituality and transpersonal psychology continues to grow including within professions such as psychiatry, psychology and counselling and for clinicians belonging to different therapeutic organisations such as Eye Movement Desensitisation and Reprocessing (EMDR) therapy.

Let me explain what I mean by 'spirituality' in HLP. I think this is an important point to establish early on, because people have different views and opinions and this can make it extremely difficult to find a unanimous agreement on a definition.

The *Oxford Dictionary* defines spirituality as:

> The quality of being concerned with the human spirit or soul as opposed to material or physical things.

Teilhard de Chardin, a French idealist philosopher and Jesuit priest, described us as spiritual beings that have human experiences. Daniel Sulmasy, a medical doctor and philosopher, referred to spirituality as:

> An individual's or a group's relationship with the transcendent, however that may be construed. Spirituality is about the search for transcendent meaning. Most people express their spirituality in religious practice. Others express their spirituality exclusively in their relationship with nature, music, the arts, or a set of philosophical beliefs or relationships with friends and family.
>
> (Sulmasy, 2002, p. 25)

Like Sulmasy, HLP encourages spirituality to be all-embracing and inclusive and doesn't segregate any particular religious beliefs. Instead, it is open to the acceptance that there is something beyond the physical, cognitive and emotional experiences in this present situation and lifetime. In Buddhism, this is sometimes referred to as a consciousness. Others refer to this as God, Buddha, Mohammad, Cosmic Christ, Spirit, etc. The Brahmins refer to Brahma, a Hindu god that is deemed 'the creator' and associated with knowledge, the creative aspect of the universe and the beginning of existence. In other words, it is the Divine spark residing deep within all of us (Atman) and not the body/ego that is synonymous with the Brahma. Siegel (2017) referred to a Divine energy or Divine cosmic consciousness from above, which can be integrated with energy from Earth and the Divine essence or souls within individuals. We are possibly all referring to the same thing, just with different terminologies.

In reference to spirituality, I personally believe in a Divine Source that is the true source or energy of infinite unconditional love and that when our soul, or our Divine essence, aligns with and embraces the Divine Source, we have the potential to reach a place of bliss, sovereignty, authenticity and live our Dharma. There are many ancient and Indian religious meanings of Dharma and no single-word translation exists. Wayne Dyer has publicly spoken and written extensively about Dharma as being where everything in life has a purpose. He referred to Dharma as what you live by, an inner calling within one's heart, which becomes clear when you truly align yourself with the Divine Source (Dyer, 2013). People have reported different ways to connect with their own personal spiritual faith, for example through meditation, faith, prayer, healing, our environment and nature, music, poetry and literature, art, people, and relationships.

Being open to everything

I do not define myself as belonging to a particular religion or group. I have certainly experimented throughout my life in the search of finding a group or organisation that fits with my belief system. I was brought up in the Catholic faith and this continued to be a big part of my life until I went to university. As my spirituality widened and I questioned some of the Catholic viewpoints, I tried other religions and spiritualist and meditation groups. I do believe that there can be a great deal of comfort and support in belonging to a particular church or spiritual group, especially in times of need or distress. However, despite this, I have recently found my peace in accepting that there isn't one group or organisation that encapsulates my spiritual understanding; perhaps this allows me to remain open to the variety of beliefs different individuals have. I have also noticed that I have had spiritual experiences not only through meditation but also through contact with certain individuals, nature, places, and activities, for example, dancing, gardening, and yoga.

I am open to the belief in God, Jesus, angels, and archangels, Buddha, all of the Ascended Masters (spiritually enlightened beings who underwent spiritual transformations during their incarnations as humans) who have gone before us, as well as many other belief systems too. So, if I am working with someone who believes in God, I am comfortable utilising their own beliefs in the work we do if appropriate. The same applies to someone who may be Muslim or Buddhist or aligned with other faiths. As long as I am open to working with their belief system and hold on to the basic principles of acting in a loving, compassionate manner, I can work with whatever anyone brings. This doesn't preclude me from working with someone who has no spiritual belief system, as I don't see it as my role to try and convert individuals to any point of view. We are all permitted our own beliefs and I am highly respectful of this. I have to hold on to the position of being accepting and open, and when appropriate, curious in gaining an understanding of a client's spirituality and beliefs without judgement or criticism. I always work with what is true to them.

The soul

Spirituality can, but doesn't have to, believe in the presence of a soul, although I personally do believe in this. Again, like spirituality, it is difficult to scientifically prove or find a universally accepted definition of a soul. However, there is an understanding within the many different religions and philosophical studies that a soul is an incorporeal essence of a living being. In the *Collected Works of The Mother* (Mother, 1972, p. 247), the soul is defined as:

> The divine spark that dwells at the centre of each being; it is identical with its Divine Origin; it is the Divine in man.

In his description of soul-centred psychotherapy, Powell (2018, p. 73) refers to the soul as 'the manifestation of spirit through form,' suggesting that everything has a soul, but that humans are more advanced to include self-consciousness or '*awareness of awareness.*' Tomlinson (2012) refers to the soul as a pure spirit energy, which holds all the memories and experiences from each incarnation. For me, the soul is an immortal, invisible energy, the Divine within us that originated from the Divine Source of unconditional love. I believe the soul is connected to our higher selves and carries our infinite memories, experiences and knowledge.

If the reader would like to explore more about a soul's journey then I would recommend Newton's *Journey of Souls* (2011) and subsequent publications by the same author. Like Newton, I see myself first and foremost as a soul. In essence, I believe I am a soul first that is housed in a physical body that has emotions, sensations, and beliefs. In this lifetime I happen to be a female, but that doesn't mean that I have always been reincarnated as a female. I believe my soul holds all the information and memories of my past lives as well as challenges and traumas that I have experienced. Believing in a soul, or the concept of reincarnation however, is not essential nor is it a pre-requisite for working spiritually with individuals.

Exploring spirituality within yourself

If you are interested in using a spiritual approach with your clients, it is important for you to be open to the concept of spirituality and be comfortable in your own beliefs without feeling the need to force these onto anyone else. If you are new to the topic of spirituality and interested in discovering how to live a more spiritual life, I would highly recommend watching Wayne Dyer's film called *The Shift*. It portrays how to live a more authentic life and how opportunities can present themselves to open up to this concept. This is a lovely film to recommend to clients too.

Spiritual questions to explore within yourself

Below are some important questions to ask YOURSELF before starting this work with your clients. If you are used to meditating then this can also be a process you can use to discover your answers and notice how they make you feel. There are no right or wrong answers to any of these questions, just observe what is true to you at this given stage in your life journey. Explore these questions with an openness and acceptance and without judgement or criticism of yourself and others.

1   How would you define your spiritual beliefs?
2   Did you grow up in a spiritual or religious environment? Are you still involved with those spiritual or religious traditions or views today or have they changed, and if so in what way?
3   What are the spiritual or religious views of your parents or significant people in your life?
4   How do other people's spiritual beliefs impact on you?
5   Do you believe in the concept of a soul?
6   From a spiritual level, what do you believe happens when people die?
7   Do you believe in past lives?
8   What is your understanding of why we are here?
9   Do you believe there is a higher source of unconditional love or energy that we all have the potential to align with if we choose?
10 Do you believe in spiritual guides, guardians, angels, archangels, etc.?
11 How have your spiritual beliefs impacted on your daily life and journey so far?
12 Do you believe that we meet people during a lifetime in order to learn, teach or heal one another?
13 Do you believe that everything happens for a reason or that there are just coincidences or luck?
14 Do you feel that you want to be able to achieve things but feel a block in the way of doing this?
15 Do you live life through your heart and/or soul or through your ego?
16 Do you find yourself getting into repeated patterns of behaviour with situations or other people?

17 Are you able to identify something positive within a challenge you experience?
18 Are you busy 'doing' rather than 'being'?
19 Do you meditate or nurture yourself or practice self-care?
20 Do you find it easy to be compassionate and non-judgemental to yourself and others?

As you ask yourself these questions, try to adopt a level of self-enquiry and curiosity to this process, identifying any held unconscious biases that you may be holding, including those that may be related to your social identity (sex, gender, race, culture, age, social class, or religion), your world views and experiences, any generational/ancestral trauma and learning as well as experiences you have had, or people you have encountered in your own life. The more understanding you have about yourself and the more experience you have on your own spiritual journey, the more open and receptive you will be to others. As your confidence and spiritual understanding in exploring these questions within yourself increases, so will your intuition on how best to tailor the topic to your client. One possible way of developing this confidence is to try asking your friends what their spiritual views and ideas are. This may help you to work out whether certain beliefs trigger anxiety or discomfort in you, or whether your interest and passion are stimulated.

Exploring spirituality with your client

As your own spiritual awareness increases, so will your ability to identify signs or opportunities with clients that allow the topic of spirituality to open up. Practising mindfulness will strengthen your awareness within clinical work and this is discussed in Chapter 4. Mindfulness practice has been reported to increase a sense of trust and closeness with others (Kabat-Zinn, 1994). Daniel Siegel (2010) suggested that engaging in mindfulness allows therapists to attune and resonate with their clients. Therapists using mindfulness have been shown to bring these skills into their clinical work, which can strengthen the therapeutic relationship (Aggs & Bambling, 2010). Siegel (2013) conducted a heuristic research study investigating the impact of spiritual resonance between therapists and clients in order to explore the energetic interaction that can occur. She described spiritual resonance as:

> Vibrational patterns of greater cosmic wholeness experienced through soul awareness; inclusive of all forms of resonances; not component based; and transmitted multidirectionally in the energy field between therapist, client, Divine Source, and Earth.

(2013, p. 49)

During the process of resonance, it is suggested that one moves beyond the egoic mind to access a higher presence, cosmic energy, or Divine force, which can be very transformative and healing when working with clients. If you are interested in exploring a spiritual journey, or perhaps you are already embarking along this path, you may start noticing your intuition develop, this may take the form of physical sensations, a sense of knowing, inner hearing and seeing. These are all symptoms that I have experienced and that have also been reported elsewhere (e.g. Braud & Anderson, 1998; Siegel, 2013; Dent, 2025).

Siegel (2018) advocated that the aim of a transpersonal therapist is to help individuals go beyond the healing of their trauma through an awakening process so that they can achieve their highest potential. A transpersonal therapist aims to work with an open heart and soul, connecting with their true authentic self as they support the client through the different stages of awakening. This may include exploration of all aspects of life, the world and their existence, for example, 'Who or what am I?' and 'What is the meaning of life?' The transpersonal therapist does not view the client as fundamentally different from themselves. Instead, they acknowledge the completeness within their client, even if the client is initially unable to recognise this with themselves.

The more familiar you are with exploring your own beliefs, the more comfortable you will feel about doing this with others. Clients can be vulnerable and it is imperative that we never take advantage of this by forcing or inflicting our ideas or beliefs on to them. You can use any of the questions that you have been asking yourself with your clients, but try not to overdo this; only explore areas that are pertinent to the work that you may feel will benefit them and that are relevant to them rather than asking just for the sake of asking or enforcing your belief system onto the client. Working in a spiritual way is much the same as any other psychological work we do. The aim is to adopt Socratic questioning that keeps the dialogue open and curious. A simple and effective question to start the process of enquiry is usually:

'I was wondering what your spiritual beliefs are?'

If you are unsure about what they have said, ask them to elaborate further. There is no harm in saying:

'Please could you tell me what you mean?'

or

'I am not familiar with that but I am really interested to learn, please could you tell me more?'

At the most this can open up an interesting and significant discussion about their spiritual beliefs, at the very least it will do no harm. They may respond by saying:

'Well I am an atheist, I don't believe in a God and don't care what happens to me when I die.'

If they do, you'll have a pretty good idea that they are not going to be interested in exploring any further spiritual discussions or be open to there being a higher source at this stage. It is, however, important to acknowledge their views as true to them. It is not your role to try and convince them otherwise. So, a simple comment may be:

'Thank you for sharing and being honest, that is really helpful to know.'

This does not mean that you cannot introduce some general concepts of spiritual work into the therapy but it will be done using a Heart Led (HL) model, which is discussed in more detail in Chapters 6 and 7, encouraging clients to live a life through their heart.

If the person responds by telling you which particular religion they belong to, this may lead on to a discussion about what their belief system is within their religion. I do not profess to be an expert on all the different types of religion and value systems and instead I try to keep an open mind and accept whatever is right for them and understand this from their perspective. Even within a particular religion people may have different beliefs and I want to remain open to this and hear their story and values. Never make assumptions because you may be wrong and this can just highlight your own prejudices and beliefs, which will interfere with this work. As with the clinical work we offer, try to see each individual as unique, with their own personal story and experiences.

Depending on how the discussion is going, and if the client shows some interest in spirituality, I usually ask whether they believe in the presence of a soul. This is allowing me to take the conversation slightly deeper, if they are interested, and will also guide me on what other healing work we could explore to complement the psychological therapy I can offer. A simple question to ask is:

'Do you believe that we have a soul?'

A person's answer to this can be very informative. If they answer 'yes' or 'maybe,' then I will ask:

'Are you open to the idea of past lives and that our soul incarnates in order to experience or gain a deeper understanding about life?'

Within all of this exploration, I am also trying to identify positive resources that are invaluable in strengthening up a person to undertake therapy, including nurturing figures, wise figures and protective figures in their current life. Examples of a spiritual support team (or wise figures) may include God, Buddha, Mohammed, many of the Hindu Gods, Angels and Archangels, and Divine Source. Even though a person may be really struggling in life and feeling very isolated, knowing that they have a spiritual support team can be hugely beneficial and if we are able to encourage them to access this during their day, it can provide strength and courage. Siegel (2017) discussed how some of her clients started awakening to their spiritual support during clinical sessions and how this could then be translated into positive internal resources.

I have so far never offended anyone by asking about their spirituality. When we go to hospital or register with GPs, dentists, or other health services, we often have to fill in questionnaires about our personal history including ethnicity, gender, and religion. I think we are more afraid to inquire about spirituality because we are unsure where to take it afterwards. It is my experience that it can play a significant part in people's lives and that not asking the question closes down a whole area of work that could be extremely powerful and helpful for the individual. I am constantly fascinated by the value of exploring spirituality with my clients and many feel relieved or interested in taking their healing to a deeper level. It is not uncommon for someone to tell me that they do have spiritual interests but that these have become shut down over time and they physically, emotionally, and spiritually light up in the room at the possibility of re-igniting this area. In this way, I am acting as a catalyst for what is already there.

Case example of identifying a spiritual support team

Jenny was a 17-year-old female who attended my clinic with her mother because she had been suffering with anxiety and panic attacks for approximately four years. She had a history of self-harm and suicidal ideation and an attempted overdose. She had seen a counsellor previously but with little success and had also been seen by Child & Adolescent Mental Health Service (CAMHS), as well as a private Child Psychiatrist and was taking anti-depressants. A detailed assessment highlighted bullying in secondary school, as well as trauma related to the illness and death of a grandparent. There was also some anxiety within the extended family history. During the assessment Jenny disclosed that she saw 'shadows' everywhere. She had recently told a counsellor at her college who had panicked and set alarm bells ringing with concerns that Jenny had hallucinations. Not surprisingly this caused Jenny further distress.

I asked Jenny a simple question – 'Do you find these shadows positive or negative?' Jenny told me that she found them positive, she wasn't afraid of them, they had always been there and on the contrary they talked to her and give her helpful advice. I explored with Jenny whether she believed these shadows could be some sort of positive or spiritual support that she was connected to. Jenny burst into tears and felt a huge sense of relief as she felt understood for the first time. Both her mother and Jenny were very emotional because they didn't feel I was judging or criticising Jenny's shadows and I also gave an explanation as to what they could possibly represent for her. We discussed how we could use these shadows as part of her spiritual support team to support her if needed with the therapy that we had planned. Jenny learned how to trust her shadows and work with them rather than believing that she had to be scared of their presence.

What if you or your clients are not spiritual?

Not every client will be open to working spiritually and that is fine. However, I believe that the key concepts from the HL model can still provide some wisdom along the way and guide people to not only understand how to handle everyday life challenges, but also how they can learn and grow from these opportunities.

Some therapists will feel uncomfortable working within a spiritual framework, but they need to be aware of whether they are hindering their client's growth because of their own belief system or fear. If a client is ready and willing for their psychotherapeutic work to embody a spiritual perspective, then surely we are doing them a disservice by not facilitating this. Referring them to a therapist who is able to facilitate and work within a spiritual dimension is just as important, as this recognises our own limitations without imposing them on our clients. I am very clear within my Clinical Psychology practice on where my strengths and weaknesses lie. It would be unethical of me to work with clients when I have little experience or knowledge in the area in which they are struggling, but I am more than willing to refer them to someone else with the expertise required.

Embarking on a spiritual journey can be an incredibly lonely and frightening experience for our clients. I cannot emphasise enough that we have to help them to move away from the spiritual idea of 'getting it,' or 'getting to the end of the spiritual journey,' or reaching an 'enlightened state' because that concept is often driven from the ego and expectations and not from the heart. Life is a journey, it is about experiencing that journey and being open to the experiences along the process. There is always so much to learn and gain by being open to receiving and if your client closes any doors they could miss out on something important. We can all learn so much from encounters with other people and situations.

What is HLP?

HLP is a spiritually informed psychotherapy that provides a way of teaching clients to start living a life through their heart and soul rather than their ego, so that they live a more authentic life, which is freer of pain and suffering. In HLP, the term 'ego' (discussed in detail in Chapter 3) is used to refer to an individual's 'self-image' or conscious perceived thoughts and over-analysis of the world in which they live, where subject and object are considered distinct and separate. The term 'heart' refers to a person's emotional centre that is the source of unconditional love, compassion, inner wisdom and truth.

The word 'psychotherapy' is derived from ancient Greek where *psyche* is the 'breath, spirit or soul' and *therapeia* is 'healing.' HLP therefore encapsulates healing of the spirit or soul through heart led techniques that are spiritually informed.

HLP has two working models. The HL (Heart Led) model *can be used with any client regardless of their spiritual beliefs*. For many clients this is sufficient and can be used either as a standalone spiritually informed psychotherapy, or can be incorporated with other psychotherapies (discussed in Chapter 2). If clients are open to

Challenges, trauma and attachment difficulties

Blocks and restrictions

Repeated themes or patterns of

behaviour/situations

EGO   EGO

Psychological difficulties

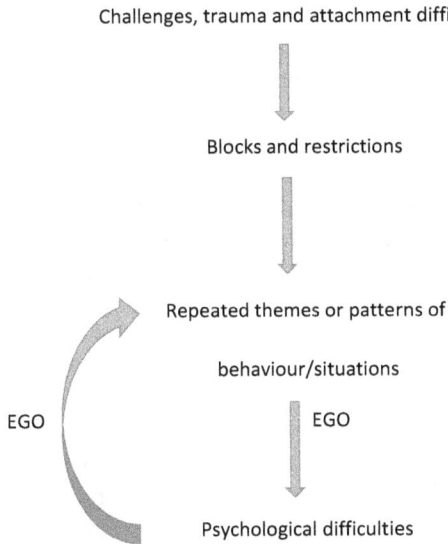

Figure 1.1 Underpinnings of HLP

spirituality then the HASL (Heart and Soul Led) model supports clients to honour what feels authentic at a soul level as well as a heart level.

The process of applying HLP with clients is discussed in Part 3. Both models have the same underpinnings, which support the understanding of the root cause of a client's psychological distress and are illustrated in Figure 1.1. To summarise:

- Challenges, trauma, or attachment/relationship difficulties create blocks and restrictions.
- Blocks and restrictions cause repeated themes or patterns of behaviour/situations.
- The repeated themes lead to psychological distress. The ego creates a repetitive cycle that maintains the repeated themes.

In the context of this book, the word trauma is used to represent any life event or repeated enduring events that have caused significant distress and has interfered with an individual's ability to cope with normal functioning. Examples include: bullying, attachment issues, abuse (sexual, physical, verbal, and neglect), accidents or illnesses, and many other situations where a person has felt that they did not have a sense of safety or being in control, or where they felt responsible or self-defective in situations. Traumatic symptoms can manifest hours, weeks, months, or years after the event.

Key concepts of HLP

The key concepts behind HLP are based on some spiritually informed beliefs (rather than proven facts). This includes the idea that life is seen as an individual journey in which there are opportunities to understand and experience life lessons. Weiss and Weiss (2012) suggested that souls incarnate to learn spiritual lessons that once achieved mean reincarnation is no longer needed. By gaining a higher perspective of our soul's journey through many lifetimes, they suggested that we are able to release guilt, despair, and a sense of feeling trapped or being rushed and instead embrace the journey. They believed that the intuitive knowledge gained from understanding our soul's journey can help clear many obstacles that may have been indoctrinated during our lifetimes, allowing us to recognise ourselves as a loving spiritual being so that we can attain our highest potential and heal ourselves and the world we live in. Weiss and Weiss (2012) discussed how transformation can occur by multi-dimensional healing from past life memories at a physical, spiritual and emotional level. They and other past life regression therapists (e.g. Newton, 2011; Tomlinson, 2012) have suggested we come back time and time again to work within soul groups on our individual spiritual journeys, facilitating each other in the process by deciding who will play each character in a particular lifetime, for example, parent, sibling, child, partner or lover, friend. Through reincarnation, challenging relationships present themselves as chances to heal and forgive any difficulties that have arisen between souls in past lives and interactions create opportunities to learn, teach or heal within or between souls.

Key concepts of the HL model

- Everyone is on their own individual life journey.
- The life journey is an opportunity to experience life lessons. Life lessons are themes to experience that provide opportunities to honour the authentic self.
- Encounters with other individuals offer opportunities to learn, teach, or heal oneself or others.
- Each individual has a primary life lesson and sometimes a few secondary life lessons to experience.
- Primary and secondary life lessons may be specific to certain areas of a person's life or more general. Areas that can be affected include: work, finances, significant relationships, health, personal growth, spirituality, friendships, family, hobbies and interests, environment, or systems.
- Individuals may have a number of joint life lessons with a few significant individuals in their life where they can work together on an additional theme from their primary life lesson.
- Everyday and systemic life lessons provide additional opportunities to experience life lessons.
- All challenging experiences, relationships, or traumas are opportunities to experience life lessons.
- Within each challenge there is a choice to be made. Making new choices that do not repeat patterns is essential for life lessons to be fully experienced. Making new choices is extremely difficult.
- The ego is the biggest barrier to making new choices.

- Psychological distress can result when choices are made that are ego driven.
- If a choice is made that doesn't enable the life lesson to be understood, then another challenge with a similar theme will occur and these challenges will be represented as repeated patterns in a person's life. This continues until a thorough understanding is made of the primary life lesson.
- Choices made from the heart lead to better outcomes and gain wisdom in life lessons.
- Making heart led choices sometimes requires a leap of faith, venturing into new territory without knowing what the outcome will be. When a leap of faith is taken, progress is made with the individual's life lesson/s.
- Making heart led choices allows an individual to express themselves more authentically and live a life with more ease and grace.

Additional key concepts of the HASL model

All of the above key concepts of the HL model are applied to the HASL model, but at a soul level this is taken one step further.

- When created, each soul was perfectly aligned with the Divine Source.
- Each soul decided which life lesson/s it would like to experience as a theme. Life lessons are extremely challenging and a soul may spend many lifetimes experiencing their lessons.
- Souls work within a primary soul group interacting in a complex way, so that souls collectively facilitate each other to experience their own individual life lessons through different encounters and challenges. Joint lessons are part of this experience but the main aim is to help each individual soul experience their primary (and secondary) life lesson.
- Before each incarnation, souls choose who will take the significant role as each of the main family members (mother, father, siblings, and children). It is like creating a script for a drama and different souls from the primary soul group will decide which character they will play, and the basis of the different scenes. During another incarnation, the roles may be completely different but the basic principle remains the same – each soul is provided with an opportunity to experience their own life lesson by learning, teaching and healing as well as facilitating other souls.
- Other soul groups interact and facilitate each other and can help each other out by acting as a 'stand-in' or an 'extra part' to facilitate other souls in their life lessons. Therefore, not every incarnation is a major learning opportunity for each soul – some will have the lead roles in the play or scene while others will be 'extras.'
- Souls do not experience difficult challenges in order to be punished or because they are lacking or bad in some shape or form. At a soul level, they choose what they would like to experience and the circumstances required. For example, if someone is blind in a particular incarnation, it doesn't mean that they must have

done something bad in previous lifetimes. On the contrary, their soul would have chosen this so that as a human being they can experience life without sight to enable them to utilise their other senses more fully to experience their life lesson. It just gives their soul a different perspective to have that experience in a particular incarnation.

- During different lifetimes, situations may happen that create blocks and restrictions at a soul level – usually when a soul (incarnated as an individual in that lifetime) has been forced or has forced another soul to do something against their wishes.
- Soul blocks and restrictions make it harder for the soul to align with the Divine Source and cause suffering and pain that can result in psychological distress.
- Soul blocks and restrictions can occur not only at an individual soul level but also between different souls, which explains why some relationships are particularly difficult.
- Most soul blocks and restrictions are carried into the next incarnation. This makes it even harder for the soul to experience their life lessons.
- A soul continues to reincarnate until it decides it has understood the primary life lesson sufficiently (this does not always mean a completion of a life lesson). A soul may then change themes and find the value of experiencing another life lesson.
- Soul level healing can clear past life blocks and restrictions so that a soul can more freely experience life lessons and make new choices.
- Making heart and soul led choices is essential for the soul's life lessons to be experienced. Even when blocks and restrictions have been removed at a soul level, a soul may continue to make ego led choices, thus repeating past behaviours and remaining stuck. However, this is now a conscious choice.
- Making heart and soul led choices often requires leaps of faith. The Divine Source will provide all that is needed to make the leap successful thus resulting in a more positive outcome.
- Souls can choose to move away from the Divine Source into darkness, instead drawing their energy from the environment (situations, places, and people). Such souls are likely to cause harm and suffering to others. At any point souls always have the choice of re-aligning with the Divine Source and be a vessel for unconditional love.

While the above additional key concepts of the HASL model are based on the belief that a soul reincarnates, these may not be compatible with some individuals understanding or belief system about a soul. Some clients may believe in a soul that is just present in this lifetime and that is okay, because ultimately the idea is to work with that resonates with your client. If they are comfortable with the concept of a soul but not the idea of past lives or incarnation, you can still work with clients using HLP, guiding them to start living a heart and soulful life but just omit reference to past lives or soul level healing.

Summary

- Key contributors to the field of transpersonal psychotherapy have explored how altered states of consciousness can transcend the ego, time and space, and empirical reality to facilitate a connection with a Divine force, adopting a non-dualistic approach to their work.
- A transpersonal psychotherapy approach evolved as a branch of psychology in the 1960s and 1970s to take into account reported spiritual, mystical, and transformative experiences that are 'beyond' the individual.
- Jung's incorporation of different archetypes, including the Persona, Self, Shadow, and Anima/Animus have been very influential in understanding aspects of the spiritual process.
- There are different forms that spiritual awakening can take including: a sudden awakening (perhaps through a significant life event or trauma), a more gradual awakening over time, Kundalini awakening, NDE, spiritual crisis, or emergency.
- New ways of connecting to the quantum field as part of a spiritual journey are currently being explored.
- Spirituality can be referred to as the ability to be open to the acceptance that there is something beyond the physical, cognitive and emotional experiences in this present situation and lifetime. It may include the belief in a higher source, which I have referred to as Divine Source (a universal source of unconditional love) as well as the presence of a soul.
- Before discussing spirituality with your clients, it is important for you as a therapist to reflect and understand your own beliefs.
- Being open to and accepting of spirituality enables clinicians to work with clients whatever their belief system in a non-judgemental manner. Never try to force your client to have the same beliefs as you – accept what is true to them.
- Keep an eye out for any indications that may suggest your client is spiritually aware. Sometimes this can be found in activities they participate in, for example, yoga, Tai Chi, meditation or mindfulness, retreats, attending church or spiritualist groups.
- HLP is informed by certain spiritually held beliefs where life is considered an individual journey in which life lessons are themes to experience and provide opportunities to honour the authentic self.
- Challenges happen in order to help individuals experience life lessons, as well as learn, teach or heal themselves and/or others.
- HLP provides two models. The HL model works within a current life domain and supports clients to live a heart led life. It identifies how psychological issues are the result of trauma and attachment difficulties that lead to blocks and restrictions, which result in repeated themes or patterns of behaviour or situations. The HL model then guides clients through a process to break out of the repeated themes and start living a heart led life. The HL model can be used with anyone regardless of their spiritual beliefs.

- If your client is open to spirituality and the presence of a soul, then the HASL model can be utilised. The HASL model has the same underlying key concepts as the HL model, but also includes ways to support clients to live a heart and soul led life as well as incorporating possible soul level healing.
- If your client is open to the concept of a soul but the idea of past lives or reincarnation does not resonate with them, you can still use HLP. The simplest way to do this would be using the HL model where you would refer to 'heart and soul' rather than just 'heart.'

2

BioPsychoSocioSpiritual approach to treating psychological distress

You have to grow from the inside out. None can teach you, none can make you spiritual. There is no other teacher but your own soul.

Swami Vivekananda

This chapter discusses how HLP can provide spiritually informed psychotherapy as part of a BioPsychoSocioSpiritual model in treating psychological distress. Using a BioPsychoSocioSpiritual approach, I describe how HLP can be offered: either as a standalone therapy or incorporated with other psychotherapies if required. In particular, one such psychotherapy that works very well in combination with HLP is the trauma-based therapy Eye Movement Desensitisation and Reprocessing (EMDR), and details are provided about how this is achieved to enable multi-dimensional healing. The chapter concludes with a discussion on when to introduce HLP to clients: either during the assessment phase, or once treatment has commenced, and case studies are provided to illustrate how this can be achieved.

The development of a BioPsychoSocioSpiritual Model

Engel (1977) initially proposed adopting a BioPsychoSocial model in medicine and psychiatry that was revolutionary at the time, as it was moving away from the previous linear cause-and-effect mentality to allow the integration of psychosocial factors. Therefore, within this model, some of a client's difficulties may be biologically based, that is, as a result of a chemical imbalance (often genetic) and in such instances medical intervention may be the most appropriate treatment. Difficulties may also be psychological in nature, often identifying the impact of attachment relationships throughout their life, as well as significant life events or traumas experienced. In addition, understanding the social situations and environment that a client has experienced, or is currently inhabiting, is imperative when determining how much these have impacted, or are still impacting on their life, experiences, and choices. It is not uncommon to see someone who is feeling affected by a negative or toxic work situation, school environment, or home life, where changes using a social or systemic framework can lead to psychological improvement.

DOI: 10.4324/9781003613749-3

One of the main reasons why clients enter therapy is because they are dissatisfied with various aspects of their lives or because they are suffering and in pain and seek relief from this discomfort. It is our role as therapists and clinicians to facilitate clients in finding relief using a variety of different psychological, systemic, and biological techniques and interventions depending on our experience and training. By adopting a BioPsychoSocial model, wonderful healing can come from utilising many of the psychotherapies currently available. For example, EMDR (Shapiro, 2018) is a very effective trauma therapy that processes distressing memories into adaptive resolution and I am always impressed at how individuals can reach a place of healing by finding compassion, forgiveness, or acceptance when using this therapy. Dyadic Developmental Psychotherapy (DDP) is another powerful intervention which uses an approach that incorporates playfulness (representing a lightness and sense of hope), acceptance, curiosity, and empathy (known as PACE), to engage and work deeply with very traumatised, abused, or neglected individuals (Hughes, 2007; Golding, 2008), although it is also a wonderful way of engaging with any client regardless of their attachment history. Some psychotherapies are particularly focused on acceptance, for example, Acceptance and Commitment Therapy (Hayes, Strosahl, & Wilson, 2016) or Mindfulness. Most traditional psychotherapies, however, tend to focus on the present life domain and do not take into account spirituality or potential past life issues and trauma. Incorporating a spiritual intervention can complement and enhance our current skills and expertise.

Some authors began to recognise the importance of including spirituality within healthcare provisions (McKee & Chappel, 1992; King, 2000), but it was Sulmasy (2002) who proposed a philosophical anthropology to a BioPsychoSocioSpiritual model when treating clients at the end of their lives, where spirituality is considered intrinsic within the individual. Since then, a BioPsychoSocioSpiritual approach has been explored more widely, including the areas of health psychology, family therapy, chronic pain, and cancer. Taking this one step further, Hacker Hughes (2017) suggested that a BioPsychoSocioSpiritual approach could be used to understand psychological distress including anxiety, depression, and Post Traumatic Stress Disorder (PTSD). His experience is similar to mine in that the traditional BioPsychoSocial approach does not consider everything in a person's life because it omits the opportunity to address how a spiritual perspective can provide an understanding of psychological distress and deeper healing if desired. Read (2019) proposed a BioPsychoSocialArchetypal approach when working with clients, influenced by Carl Jung's concept of the archetype. Taking a similar philosophy, Dobo (2023) provided a framework to integrate Jungian psychology within EMDR therapy. Internal Family Systems (IFS) therapy, developed by Schwartz in the 1980s, is a great example of how spirituality can play a significant role in the therapy and healing process (Schwartz, 2023). I have also written in detail about incorporating a spiritual and energetic perspective into EMDR therapy throughout all stages of the EMDR process (Dent, 2025), illustrating how a BioPsychoSocioSpiritual model can benefit anyone regardless of what stage they are on during their life journey.

Psychological distress

Initial assessment

BioPsychoSocial model   ⟷   BioPsychoSocioSpiritual model

Heart Led Psychotherapy

(Heart Led model or Heart and Soul Led model)

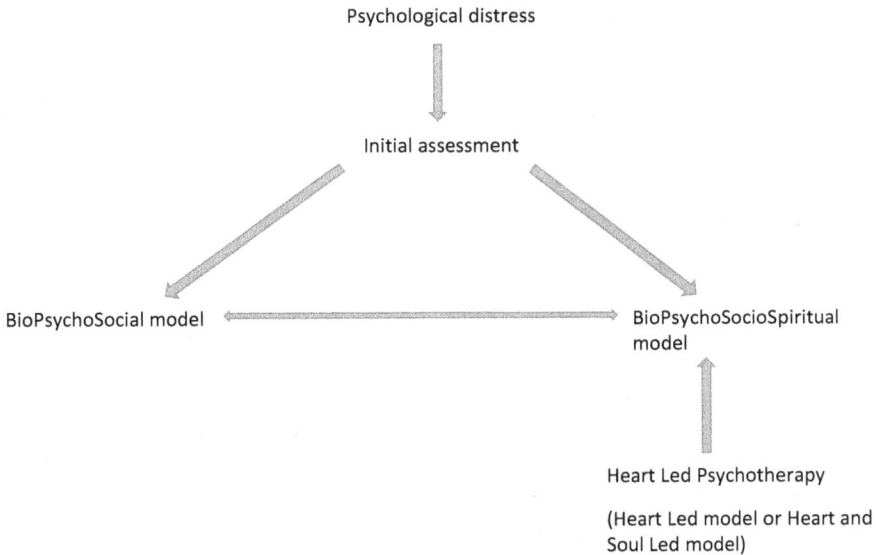

Figure 2.1 Heart Led Psychotherapy as part of a BioPsychoSocioSpiritual approach

HLP as part of a BioPsychoSocioSpiritual model

HLP can provide a spiritually informed therapy in a BioPsychoSocioSpiritual model when treating psychological distress, and this is illustrated in Figure 2.1.

The key to offering HLP within a BioPsychoSocioSpiritual approach is to identify clients' challenges, traumas, and attachment issues, along with resulting blocks and restrictions that have caused repeated themes in a client's history and which have culminated in psychological distress (previously illustrated in Figure 1.1 in Chapter 1). The first stage is to complete an initial assessment with your client and determine whether they would benefit from either:

1   *BioPsychoSocial intervention*

This would be using traditional psychotherapies either because the client is not interested or willing to explore a spiritual component to their difficulties, or because there does not appear to be a necessity to add a spiritual component (usually when the symptoms are fairly minor, the client has an uncomplicated background history and there are no obvious indications of blocks and restrictions or repeated themes). An example of this is with a client I saw who presented with an uncomplicated background history, no particular spiritual beliefs, secure attachments but was struggling to come to terms with a friend's death, which was impacting on his mood and ability to engage at work. It was possible to resource this client and use EMDR to process the grief which improved his mood and engagement at work and no further input was required. Similarly, you may have clients who present with single traumatic events (for example a road traffic accident) or younger clients who may come with minor bullying or school-based issues. I suspect the likelihood of seeing such straightforward cases now is minimal, as most clients who present to services have much more complicated and entrenched histories.

2   BioPsychoSocioSpiritual intervention

This intervention incorporates the additional spiritual framework in therapy and the majority of clients who seek support will have a history where the concepts of HLP can be applied. The HL model will look at current life difficulties but does not make reference to past lives or the soul. This can be beneficial in increasing clients' awareness of their circumstances, as well as giving them tools to make new heart led choices and reduce the repeated themes that have been keeping them stuck. If a client believes in the concept of a soul, the HASL model can be utilised. HLP can be applied as a standalone therapy within a BioPsychoSocioSpiritual approach or in conjunction with other psychotherapies. For example, if a client has a traumatic history, then HLP can provide a spiritual understanding of their difficulties, but they may also need additional therapies to process traumatic events. EMDR is a particularly useful trauma-based therapy to use in conjunction with HLP and this is discussed below and case studies are provided in Chapter 10 to illustrate how this works in practice.

HLP offers the opportunity to provide a multi-dimensional level of healing. It does not focus purely on affect regulation, but instead adds a broader spiritual understanding to where clients are (often unknowingly) living through their egos rather than their heart and soul. It provides a pathway to understand how challenges help them to experience and understand life lessons in order to make new choices that are heart and soul led. In general, due to the complexity of clients' presentations and their openness to spirituality, I find I am increasingly working with a BioPsychoSocioSpiritual model.

EMDR

There is increasing interest in how to combine spirituality with EMDR to provide multi-dimensional healing and in my own clinical work I have recognised and written about how HLP complements EMDR when developing a package of care to heal traumas (Dent, 2025). This next section discusses how this can be achieved.

What is EMDR?

EMDR is a powerful trauma therapy originally developed by Shapiro in 1987. When a person experiences a trauma or significant life event, fragments of that memory (including images, thoughts, sensory experiences, and emotions) are believed to be frozen in time and isolated in their own neural network, held in a dysfunctional, non-adaptive, and state-specific form. This can prevent the brain from processing the memory. Connecting with an unprocessed traumatic memory, even long after the event has happened, can make a person feel as if they are still experiencing symptoms of the trauma. Although the exact mechanism is still unclear, EMDR uses an adaptive information processing (AIP) model to enable the fragments of the memory to connect to appropriate associations and be processed to an adaptive and healthy resolution (Shapiro, 2018).

EMDR consists of eight distinguishable phases: history-taking, preparation, assessment, desensitisation, installation, body scan, closure, and re-evaluation. The AIP system is activated during phase four, the desensitisation phase, using bilateral dual attention. This is when an individual is first asked to connect to the worst moment of a trauma and identify the:

- Image.
- Negative cognition.
- Positive cognition.
- Validity of the positive cognition (VOC) on a scale of 1 to 7, where 1 represents completely false and 7 represents completely true.
- Emotions.
- Subjective units of distress (SUDS) on a scale of 0 to 10 where 0 represents no disturbance and 10 represents the worst possible disturbance.
- Body location.

The therapist then uses bilateral stimulation (BLS) using eye movements, sound, or tapping to stimulate the brain from left to right, in sets, usually between 24 to 28 BLS per cycle. After each set, the client is asked to briefly describe what they noticed happen. This continues until all aspects of the memory have been processed to an adaptive resolution.

In phase five, the installation phase, the positive cognition is paired with the original memory and BLS is applied to enhance the validity of the positive belief until it is completely true (VOC is 7/7). It isn't always possible to complete the processing of a distressing memory during one session, especially if the memory is very traumatic. To make sure that the client leaves the sessions in a positive frame of mind, they are asked to connect to one of the resources they have previously learned, typically their 'safe/calm place,' which is a resource technique clients are taught in imagination, where they can connect to a place that feels safe or calm (Shapiro, 2018). Alternatively, they can be asked 'What is the most important or meaningful thing that has come out of the work we did today?' Ideally you are looking for a self-referencing positive statement that can be installed using slow BLS, allowing the client to leave the session in a calm and resourced state.

EMDR was originally developed for clients with PTSD for which there is now a wealth of literature, including randomised control trials, which illustrate the effectiveness of EMDR in treating this disorder, including recommended prevention and treatment guidelines in the International Society for Traumatic Stress Studies in 2019. Additionally, its effectiveness for healing trauma is also recognised by the World Health Organisation (2013). EMDR has also been researched and demonstrated to be an effective therapy for many different psychological difficulties, including anxiety, depression, obsessive compulsive disorder, psychosis, and much more. It can also be used with young children where developmental modifications are applied (Tinker & Wilson, 1999; Lovett, 2015). EMDR is therefore an effective therapy to treat unprocessed memories that underlie trauma or significant life events.

EMDR and transpersonal psychology

Several different authors have recognised how a spiritual component can be applied when using EMDR (for example, Parnell, 1996; Hacker Hughes, 2017; Siegel, 2017, 2018; Dent, 2025). Similarities between EDMR and Vipassana meditation were reported by Parnell (1996), particularly in relation to dual attention or awareness, as well as encouraging the client to notice whatever arises during the process without judgement. Parnell also discussed how EMDR processing and meditation facilitated clients in reaching a place of compassion and inner truth, something that I have also observed in my clinical practice. Marich and Dansiger (2017) wrote about the importance of mindfulness practice within EMDR therapy, providing practical meditation exercises to teach clients how to learn these skills. Different types of spiritual resources that can be used with clients were described by Parnell (2008), including spiritual figures, connecting with a higher power, the essential spiritual self, wise beings, and spiritual experiences and teachings, a finding consistent with Siegel (2017, 2018, 2019) and also within my clinical practice (Dent, 2025). O'Malley (2018) introduced a new groundbreaking approach, sensorimotor-focused EMDR (SF-EMDR), which also integrates many spiritual concepts to provide a holistic and multi-dimensional way to heal clients. He believes that SF-EMDR facilitates clients toward the 'path of the heart.' This is facilitated by integrating information from the gut-brain and head-brain to achieve resonance at the level of the heart-brain. O'Malley later went on to introduce the term 'Quantum EMDR' (O'Malley, 2024), incorporating ideas and research from quantum physics to support his clients to connect with the quantum field in his EMDR practice.

Parnell (1996) observed that EMDR enables some of her clients to go beyond their egos to connect with transcendent or cosmic experiences. Similar findings were reported by Siegel (2017, 2018, 2019) who researched how clients working with transpersonal EMDR therapists can experience cosmic encounters during EMDR processing including healing light, spiritual guides, or facilitators, to bring about multi-dimensional healing. She illustrated how spiritual resonance can greatly facilitate EMDR processing and the multi-dimensional, transpersonal healing of traumas. Siegel (2017, 2018, 2019) found that when experienced transpersonal therapists, who were also EMDR trained, incorporated spiritual practice into their clinical work, a positive outcome was observed. Interestingly, Parnell (2008) made reference to life lessons that can be realised through life experiences although found that they often remain unintegrated.

EMDR and spiritual interweaves

When using EMDR, the standard protocol is recommended unless there is clinical justification for using a different protocol, for example, prolonged grief, phobias, and pain (Shapiro, 2018), and this is no different when using HLP informed EMDR within a BioPsychoSocioSpiritual approach to treating trauma. Therapeutic interweaves are used if a client appears stuck or looping during EMDR processing to assist them in accessing an adaptive network. Examples of this include cognitive, educational, imaginary, or visual. Siegel (2017) applied 'cosmic' interweaves, describing this as spiritually filling the therapeutic space with Divine presence or cosmic awareness to enable her clients to connect to their higher selves, resulting in a positive shift in their belief system.

HLP informed EMDR utilises 'spiritual interweaves' when clinically justified and these include accessing spiritual guides and supporters, wise self, cosmic awareness and the Divine Source (Dent, 2025). Interweaves directly related to HLP can also be used, as long as you have explained the appropriate HLP model with your client so that they understand about life lessons and are starting to connect to and listen to their heart and soul. Different HLP spiritual interweaves are discussed in detail elsewhere (Dent, 2025) and include forming heart-to-heart connections, energy interweaves, using heart energy for intergenerational and ancestral healing, healing past lives, and clearing blocked chakras. More specific HLP interweaves include:

1 **Listening to the heart and soul**: When a client appears stuck in egoic thinking during EMDR processing, ask them to 'move into your heart or soul and listen to what your heart or soul is trying to tell you' or 'what is the message from your heart or soul?'
2 **Life lessons**: When the client appears stuck, ask them 'What do you think this challenge or situation is helping you to understand or experience?'
3 **Learning, teaching, or healing**: similar to the life lessons, when a client is stuck in processing a difficult encounter with another person then it may be helpful for you to ask your client 'what do you think this relationship is trying to help you learn, teach or heal either for yourself or them?'

Having offered a spiritual interweave, apply a set of BLS, after which you will ask your client what they notice. Most of the time you may only need to offer one spiritual interweave to get the client accessing an adaptive network so that the processing can get back on track. Sometimes it may be necessary to offer an interweave a few times as they learn to connect more at a heart or soul level, especially if the client goes back into their egoic thinking, but perseverance can prove a very effective and healing intervention.

Three-pronged approach

When Shapiro developed the EMDR standard protocol she emphasised the importance of taking a three-pronged approach by addressing the past, present, and future as part of the overall treatment package. This is firstly done by addressing past experiences that underlie the psychological issues, then working on current situations that are maintaining disturbance, and finally working on positive steps in the future (Shapiro, 2018).

HLP informed EMDR can be used during the preparation stages as well as during the desensitisation phase and it also utilises a three-pronged approach working on past, present, and future challenges. HLP recognises that past and current challenges/traumas are opportunities to experience and understand life lessons to facilitate the process of healing and this gained wisdom can then be integrated and applied to tackling future challenges. EMDR formulation of traumas often takes a clustering approach to treating traumas where similar incidents are grouped together. When one incident from each cluster is processed, this frequently has a positive generalisation effect on the other incidents in the cluster (Shapiro, 2018). While this approach would still be used, HLP formulation takes an additional broader spiritual perspective, suggesting that within traumas there will be common themes or life lessons. The advantages to using an HLP formulation alongside EMDR are that HLP not only identifies common themes amongst traumatic experiences, including whether this may be related to the client's primary life lesson, joint lesson, everyday or systemic life lessons, but that this gained knowledge can be applied during processing, enabling the client to understand the experience from a spiritually informed perspective which is more in keeping with their heart and soul. When life lessons are identified and understood, clients can gain a greater awareness and can use this knowledge not only to find resolution and acceptance of past difficulties, but also apply this to current and future challenges as they arise.

I regularly witness how clients benefit from having been taught HLP in the preparation stages of EMDR, which also helps with the processing of traumas and they can then apply this knowledge so that they are more empowered and aware to tackle future situations and challenges (Dent, 2025). It is acknowledged that future research and case studies are warranted to verify the benefits of incorporating EMDR with HLP within a BioPsychoSocioSpiritual perspective.

When to introduce HLP to your client

HLP can be introduced at any stage during the therapeutic process. When appropriate, HLP can be introduced toward the end of the initial appointment once a thorough assessment of the person's difficulties has been completed and if a good therapeutic relationship has been established where the client is feeling safe and contained. At other times, it may seem more appropriate to commence other psychological work and wait for the appropriate time. Usually, the less we try to plan for this to happen and the more open we remain as clinicians to the possibility of exploring a spiritual angle with the client's difficulties, the more favourable the outcome. This means letting go of our ego and expectations and allowing the process to unfold before us so that it becomes the perfect time for your client. I am learning to trust the process and continue to be amazed at how opportunities present themselves when I am least expecting them.

During the initial assessment

My initial assessments tend to primarily focus on establishing a good therapeutic relationship with clients while obtaining a detailed background history. I am noticing that clients are becoming increasingly aware of their repeated themes and are therefore receptive to discussing HLP very early on, even when the history-taking process is not quite complete. At this point I may introduce the basic concepts of HLP and how this can be applied to their circumstances while also making sure I complete their background history as well, so this process may extend over a few sessions.

Case example of introducing HLP during the initial assessment

Arjun was in his late 30s and was advised to come and see me by his GP because he was struggling with low mood but wanted to avoid taking medication. He was feeling overwhelmed with the increased pressures of work and family life. He identified that his main issue was his marriage and he didn't feel that he and his wife worked in partnership together, especially where their two young children were concerned. During the initial assessment, Arjun was very insightful and discussed how he felt he kept getting into repeated patterns of behaviour throughout his life. He was aware that he had always struggled to communicate his feelings to others, instead compromising and rescuing others rather than prioritising his own needs. While he was fortunate that he had experienced a supportive and loving upbringing, he was aware that he struggled to make the best of opportunities presented to him and therefore never felt he was realising his full potential. Straight away it was very evident to me that there were additional blocks and restrictions between Arjun and his wife, but also that his wife had an enmeshed relationship with members of her own biological family. Toward the end of our first appointment I was able to introduce the basics of HLP. Arjun was keen to explore this more in the following session and so once my history-taking was complete, we went through all of the stages of the HL model relating it to Arjun's circumstances. He quickly recognised how it applied to his individual life journey and was very keen to explore this model further in therapy.

During therapeutic work

There are times when HLP can be introduced after therapeutic work has commenced. You may already have recognised blocks and restrictions within your client that are causing repeated themes or dynamics in their family relations or other circumstances that suggest something more spiritual is going on, but not had the opportunity to broach this subject with them. It is therefore important to keep flexible and open to the possibility of spiritual work throughout the therapeutic process.

Case example of using HL model within a BioPsychoSocioSpiritual model once therapy has commenced – adolescent

Hardeep was a teenage client who came to see me because of low mood and trauma history. She was so resistant to therapy due to attachment issues that we first had to work on building up a good therapeutic relationship using an attachment-based model (DDP). She responded well to this and we were then able to start looking at mindfulness and other resource techniques to build up her emotional tolerance and help her become more present in life. This included a session using Ego State Therapy (Forgash & Copeley, 2008), which is particularly helpful when a person can identify different parts of their personality, for example, a self-sabotage or frightened part that are in conflict with each other and can potentially block therapeutic work. Ego State Therapy aims to integrate these parts so that the individual functions more coherently. Hardeep recognised that she had a protective part as a consequence of her past traumas, so we managed to integrate this within herself and she was then in a position to process her traumatic history using EMDR. At various stages during the therapy process, Hardeep would need time to discuss current life circumstances that were difficult for her. These particularly focused around ongoing psychological difficulties with key members of her family and the impact this had on relationships. Not only were we trying to work on her past traumas but her current life was exceptionally challenging too. I therefore introduced HLP and she readily took to this approach and was able to utilise the components of the HL model in addition to our other work.

Case example of using the HASL model within a BioPsychoSocioSpiritual model once therapy has commenced – adolescent

Hannah was a 14-year-old who was reluctantly brought to a session by her mother because of suicidal ideation. She believed that no one could help her and she had to sort things out for herself. She had made three attempts to commit suicide over the past six months, involving trying to drown herself, burn herself in a hot bath, and hang herself. All these attempts had been spontaneous rather than planned. Hannah did tell me that she didn't want to die but she didn't believe she deserved to live. She had previously seen a counsellor for six sessions but hadn't engaged well as she found the counsellor judgemental. She had also been referred to CAMHS and was placed on their waiting list but was told it could be months before any support could be offered.

In addition to writing a crisis plan, the key area I focused on was my therapeutic engagement with Hannah. At the initial appointment I was able to identify how Hannah's relationship with her father was particularly difficult; he experienced mood swings, was stressed with work, and was a binge drinker. Hannah's paternal grandfather was suspected of committing suicide when her father was 15 years old. Her paternal aunt had died 15 years previously and had lived an unhappy life, was a drinker, and had died of pneumonia.

Hannah's mother had spent many years trying to help her husband be more emotionally aware. Hannah had previously had a very close relationship with her mother. Her mother had been in a car crash when Hannah was 9 years old and Hannah had blamed herself for this. Hannah also believed the car crash caused her mother to be debilitated a few years later with fatigue, which had rendered her mother incapable of doing anything for a year, so Hannah took the blame for this too. This was an exceptionally difficult time for Hannah as her mother was not physically and emotionally available and her relationship with her father was minimal. Hannah therefore learned to shut herself down from everyone, deciding that she had to fix everything herself. She also had a history of bullying in primary school and some difficult peer friendships throughout her schooling. One of Hannah's teachers in primary school had commented about her weight, which had resulted in eating issues.

At the second session Hannah mentioned having felt a bit brighter and we completed a range of questionnaires including the Mood & Feeling Questionnaire (Angold et al., 1995; score of 44, significantly above the cut-off of 26). I then started going through some psychoeducation and she engaged well. By the third session, both Hannah and her mother reflected back how they were starting to recognise the long-term impact that Hannah's father's behaviour and inability to engage emotionally had been having on family dynamics. It was at this stage that I asked Hannah and her mother about their spiritual views. Her mother immediately responded saying she was very open to spirituality although Hannah was less enthusiastic with the concept. I asked her mother whether she believed in the presence of a soul and she confirmed that she did and started discussing how she used to do a lot of soul level healing through her Christian church, but had lost touch with this several years previously. I was curious about what work she had done and so her mother gave me some background. This led us nicely on to discussing past lives and blocks and restrictions at a soul level and the components of the HASL model. Initially Hannah was reluctant to engage, but her curiosity increased significantly as her mother and I discussed blocks and restrictions that can happen between individuals at a soul level. By the end of this session Hannah was as keen as her mother for them to explore some soul level healing. Hannah's mother was also hopeful that her husband would engage with this given that he had been actively involved with the soul work that Hannah's mother had done many years earlier. Hannah made it clear that she wanted to continue seeing me in addition to any soul healing, with the plan of teaching her mindfulness and then using EMDR to process past traumas from the bullying. Hannah's mother was very animated by the end of this third session as she felt her spirituality had been re-ignited by recognising that she already had a lot of knowledge and techniques that she could reconnect with to try and improve the home situation.

Case example of using the HASL model within a BioPsychoSocioSpiritual model once therapy has commenced – adult

Fiona was a lady in her late 20s who came with low mood. She had a history of various traumas and abusive relationships that were causing her a great deal of stress and unhappiness and impacting on her ability to maintain current relationships. During the early stages of our work I introduced her to mindfulness. This in itself was difficult because she had so far been living life in her head and thoughts. She was constantly beating herself up and judging herself and felt there was a part of her that self-sabotaged relationships. At the following session we briefly reflected on her week and she remarked that she had started being more mindful and finding the benefits of this with glimpses of peace. However, a situation had happened the night before where she had been out with friends and saw her ex-partner with another woman. This triggered distress and she reacted in a way she said she wasn't proud of and was now feeling sad and cross with herself.

I introduced the HL model to Fiona, talking about the concept of an individual life journey and encounters with others in order to learn, teach, or heal. Using the HL model, we applied the principles of HLP to her situation the night before and Fiona quickly recognised how it was an opportunity for her to practise self-compassion and self-forgiveness, something that she had always struggled with and this fitted nicely with our discussion on mindfulness a week earlier where I had introduced the idea of self-compassion. We proceeded to use Ego State work in the session where she met the part of her that she felt was her self-saboteur and she managed to reframe this part and integrate this within herself.

Interestingly a few weeks later Fiona noticed some oracle cards in my therapy room and inquired about them. I explained they can be used for guidance and it was something I used personally as part of my spiritual journey. This opened up the topic of spirituality and the presence of a soul. Fiona expressed some interest although acknowledged she didn't have much understanding. She was keen to discuss this further and before long I was sharing with her the HASL model, soul level healing and how it can complement the work we were doing. She went away to explore this option, sharing this knowledge with a close friend who was experiencing major traumas. At the next session Fiona told me that another of her close friends had been receiving spiritual guidance from my colleague, which gave Fiona the confidence to arrange an appointment herself. She was so amazed by what she learned that she went on to do some soul level healing to clear her soul level blocks and restrictions alongside the EMDR with myself where I supported Fiona to process current life traumas. Fiona responded very favourably to the combined work and reported feeling much brighter, content, at peace and that she was starting to live a more authentic life. She reported significant improvements in her relationships, work and how she handled situations.

Summary

- A BioPsychoSocial model can be applied where there is little indication that incorporating spirituality is required.
- A BioPsychoSocioSpiritual approach was initially applied when treating clients at the end of their life, but there is now growing interest to apply this more broadly when working within certain therapeutic approaches and with a range of psychological difficulties.
- Within a BioPsychoSocioSpiritual approach, HLP can be offered as the spiritual psychotherapeutic component and can be used effectively either as a standalone therapy or in combination with other psychotherapies, for example, EMDR.
- When clients are stuck in EMDR processing, spiritual interweaves can be applied including using spiritual figures, cosmic or divine awareness, and HLP informed spiritual interweaves.
- Both EMDR and HLP use a three-pronged strategy working on past, current, and future challenges. HLP understands past, current and future challenges as opportunities to learn and experience life lessons which increases clients' awareness and understanding of what these challenges represent to them on their individual journey. The greater their understanding, the more effective clients will be at managing current and future challenges.
- By keeping an open and flexible approach, HLP can be taught during any stage of the therapeutic process.

Part 2

Preparation for Heart Led Psychotherapy

3

The power of the ego

In a conflict between the heart and the brain, follow your heart.

Swami Vivekananda

An important part of HLP is recognising the significance that the ego and egoic thinking has in maintaining psychological distress and this chapter focuses on the role and power of the ego. In HLP, the ego is seen as the biggest obstacle to making new heart and soul led choices and so assisting clients to become aware of their egoic thinking early on in the therapeutic process is essential. When clients live life through their ego, they can experience suffering and pain. Choosing to live a life through their heart and soul will help them make new choices during challenges that are more in keeping with their true authentic self, develop self-love, and live a life of more ease and grace.

The ego

There are various metaphors for ego but the one I like is Eliminating God/Goodness Out:

EGO Eliminate **G**od/**G**oodness **O**ut

It is natural for therapists to worry that their clients may take offence when they discuss their ego because of its associations with narcissism and self-righteousness or self-importance. You therefore need to highlight that you are not referring to egotism; where someone strives to keep or enhance favourable views about themselves and maintain a view of self-righteousness and self-importance at the expense of others.

Over the past few centuries there has been much discussion and debate about what actually is the ego. The psychoanalytical definition of ego is:

The part of the mind that mediates between the conscious and the unconscious and is responsible for reality testing and sense of personal identity.

DOI: 10.4324/9781003613749-5

The philosophical definition of ego is:

A conscious thinking subject.

Deepak Chopra is considered an expert in the field of mind–body healing and is a world-renowned author and public speaker on alternative medicine. He suggests that the ego is our self-image instead of the authentic self:

> It is not who you really are. The ego is your self-image; it is your social mask; it is the role you are playing. Your social mask thrives on approval. It wants control, and it is sustained by power, because it lives in fear.
>
> (Chopra, 1996, p. 11)

Eckhart Tolle (2005) described the ego as one's false self, which has endless needs, creates a sense of vulnerability and fear, and attaches itself to problems. Taylor (2017) questioned some spiritual viewpoints that believe wakefulness is living a life without an ego, instead suggesting that awakened individuals may still have an ego but that it is different and one that recognises the self as an illusion. In HLP, the term ego is a term used to represent the over-thinking and over-analysis that cause suffering and distress, as well as our self-image. Learning to notice and then release egoic thinking and live life through the heart and soul may help us experience a more authentic life.

We all have been affected by our ego and if you don't believe this, then that is your ego talking! Since birth and throughout childhood we are encouraged by others; how to think, learn, have expectations, desires, and ambitions, be in control, and so forth. It is ingrained into us by the systems around us, not necessarily consciously or manipulatively but it happens nonetheless. Interestingly as the ego strengthens through our life, our awareness and ability to be mindful reduces. Sadly, children are now growing up in a culture that is dominated by social media and technology, which also impacts on the ego; they believe they have to keep up with their peer group in order to feel valued or fit in, wanting the latest technology and becoming addicted to communicating through technology rather than engaging in direct social interactions. Many children nowadays are losing their own individual identity and self-belief and most frighteningly the ability to play, be joyful, creative, free-spirited, and mindful. They and countless adults in society are hooked into technology and more research is evolving to show the detrimental impact of social technology on children's mental and psychological well-being. It is literally Eliminating God/Goodness Out!

Characteristics of the ego

- **Hooks** – the ego hooks into situations or people and clings on for dear life, causing suffering and pain. The ego strengthens the hook by justifying its necessity.
- **Expectations** – that clients have because they become dissatisfied and believe they would feel better if they achieved something or had more in their lives.

This could be in relation to others, objects and materialism – 'If I have a new car or the latest gadget then I know I am successful,' 'if I get the job then that shows I am important and significant,' 'if I had someone to love me then I would be okay.' The list is endless.

- **Victim role** – the ego persuades clients that they are still the victims in their situations long after the trauma or challenge. Therefore, it plays a central role in maintaining psychological distress because it creates a sense of powerlessness, helplessness, and vulnerability. The ego makes it hard for clients to view their situation with clarity, take ownership of the traumas or challenges, and make new choices.
- **Fear** – of being alone, unloved, or unwanted. In order to heal from this clients have to face their fear straight on and experience this to its fullest to know that they can have a love that is not dependent on anyone else, instead learning to love and accept themselves. This doesn't mean they have to spend the rest of their lives being lonely, but that when they find that place of self-love and self-worth they no longer need others to fill that void. They have filled that space with sufficient love and gratitude for whom they are, that they can live peacefully and joyously alongside others. This is a much healthier place to be, not only for themselves, but also in the relationships they have which will then complement them rather than place them in a state of dependency.

Clients' egos can easily be triggered by other people and when this activates negative emotions such as anger, hurt, frustration, or annoyance, they are more likely to respond in a confrontational, defensive, and non-compassionate manner. Learning to let go of egoic thinking is the ultimate place to be because it allows clients to be FREE – free of hooks, expectations, fear, and taking the role of a victim. Freedom from egoic thinking enables them to appreciate and enjoy everything around them. Instead of searching for what is missing in their lives, our clients start seeing and appreciating what they do have with gratitude.

I used to be quite nervous about introducing the topic of ego with clients. Now I realise that my fear was my own ego telling me that I mustn't do this because I would offend my clients! My own ego didn't want my heart and soul or anyone else's to take the lead role because it would feel redundant. I am learning that if I introduce the topic with sensitivity and compassion, I get a positive reception from clients as they readily begin to recognise how much of their lives is driven by egoic thinking, which has made them become a victim of their circumstances.

In HLP, this is how I introduce the topic of ego with my clients:

There is a general acceptance that we all have an ego. When I talk about the ego I am not referring to being narcissistic or self-righteous. Instead I am referring to that part of us that creates our thoughts and desires and expectations. Our ego is very clever, it hooks us into people or situations because it makes us believe that we need these things in order to function or survive, but this creates dependency and we stop believing that we can function without such things. Our ego makes us judge and feel judged or criticised, makes us take the blame for difficulties or feel responsible for everyone else's happiness except our own. The problem is that when we live life through our ego we often end up repeating patterns of behaviour or situations and this makes us feel stuck and trapped. We are never happy with what we do have because we are always searching for something else. Our ego doesn't want to be ignored so it provides very good arguments as to why we should stay stuck in challenging or difficult circumstances. Our ego creates FEAR about change, convincing us that something bad will happen if we make new choices – this is its biggest weapon.

When a person has many negative beliefs they tend to self-sacrifice, staying in difficult situations, believing they are deserving of this or lack self-worth. They justify this behaviour to themselves and stay stuck. However, it is their ego that is keeping them stuck by over-analysing and reinforcing the dilemma to justify to themselves and others about why the situation stays the same. One of the reasons people stay in difficult situations is that they don't believe they or others would cope if they were not around either practically, emotionally, or financially. The ego is very clever; it can create scenarios so elaborate and extreme that clients become fearful of significant change.

Although working spiritually does not necessarily require attachment to any particular religion or philosophy, there are overlaps with some major religious and spiritual teachings, for example, the Four Noble Truths in Buddhism, which can be simplified as:

1 Suffering exists.
2 Suffering arises from attachment to desires.
3 Suffering ceases when attachment to desire ceases.
4 Freedom of suffering is possible by practising the Eightfold Path (which includes right view, right intention, right speech, right action, right livelihood, right effort, right mindfulness, and right concentration).

The second Noble Truth is really explaining what happens when individuals live life through their ego – suffering is the result of attachment to something or someone (desires) and expectations. In order to stop the suffering, it is necessary to let go of these attachments and expectations (third Noble Truth), in other words, letting go of the ego.

How to teach clients to let go of their egoic thinking

- The first stage is to help clients recognise when they are listening to their ego. This requires awareness. Without awareness they will continue to listen and live by the stories the ego creates. Teaching clients mindfulness increases their awareness of when they are in the 'thinking' mode and this is discussed in more detail in Chapter 4.
- Help clients to identify what they are hooked into that is causing their suffering. Examples include holding on to an unhappy or abusive relationship, job, or living environment. Clients can also become addicted to food, money, alcohol,

drugs, or excessive exercise. There are so many situations or relationships that clients can hook into, each of which will cause suffering. Once hooks have been identified, the next stage is to support the client to LET GO OF THE HOOK. Exercise 1 below demonstrates how this can be achieved.

- Encourage clients to recognise how expectations can create blocks because once a goal has been reached they will start to question 'Now what?' Living by expectations stops clients from appreciating what they have in any given moment, instead always feeling dissatisfied and wanting something else.

- Increase clients' awareness of when they have experienced challenges and have adopted the victim role. Show clients how being the victim creates negative thinking that is really coming from their ego, which keeps them stuck and causes them to repeat themes in their life. Help clients to recognise how it makes them feel emotionally when they maintain the victim role and how this consequently then impacts on their corresponding behaviour.

- Make clients aware and accept that their ego will reveal itself from time to time, acting as a catalyst to help them learn a life lesson. The quicker they recognise when the ego appears due to their reaction to a situation or person, the quicker they can move out of the head and into their heart and soul to experience the life lesson. Exercise 2 below explains how to facilitate this process.

- Support clients to have gratitude for life challenges by understanding that something good may come from every situation however difficult that may be. Challenges present opportunities to experience important lessons that can then become gifts.

Exercise 1

Letting go of hooks

This is an exercise I was taught while on a mindfulness retreat with the Happy Buddha. Ask your client to imagine that a situation or person that they are hooked into is metaphorically resting in the palm of their hands within tightly grasped fingers. The tight grasp of their fingers represents the hook into the situation or person. Ask your client to explore what this feels like with their grasp tightly in place and notice whether they are experiencing suffering and pain anywhere in their bodies.

Now ask your client to imagine slowly releasing their grip, relaxing the fingers one at a time. Guide them in the release of their grip until they can just imagine that situation or person resting on the palm of their hand, balancing there. Again, explore with your client what this feels like now that their grasp has loosened. Has the suffering diminished? You may decide to spend a few minutes with your client supporting them in oscillating between tightening and then loosening their grip and noticing any changes in how this makes them feel.

Encourage your client to start being more aware during their day of when they notice any suffering and when they notice this happening, ask them to become aware of how tight their grip has become to the situation or people involved. Encourage your client to gently loosen their grip, observing whether the suffering eases.

Exercise 2

Ego versus heart conversation

In sessions, when you notice that the client is getting stuck with their ego or thoughts, a helpful exercise can be to first ask them if they can identify what their ego is saying to them. Then guide your client to move into their heart and ask for a response from their heart. Oscillate between the ego and heart for as long as required for the client to recognise the difference between the ego and heart messages.

Case example of ego versus heart conversation

Simon had just finished relaying his life story to me and it was very apparent that his repeated theme was being addicted to his work at the expense of his family. This was driven by an underlying belief that he needed to succeed financially to prove his self-worth. He had a deep sense of failure from early experiences in his childhood so had learned to immerse himself in his work to prove to himself and others that he could achieve and be successful in life. At the age of 53 years he sought psychological help following the advice of his GP. Two years earlier he had suffered a pulmonary embolism and nearly died. This experience left him feeling very anxious but also disconnected from everything around him (he described this as a numb feeling). When I first saw him, he had just moved out of the family home and was on the verge of a breakdown. His goals were to find a middle balance between work and home, to understand what life was about and to learn to manage his anxious feelings.

During the first session Simon was open to exploring a spiritual perspective to his difficulties, which included discussing his ego and the impact it was having on his life and the decisions he was making. In the third session, we listened to what Simon's ego was saying and then I asked him to move into his heart and notice what it was trying to communicate with him. I then asked him to let his ego respond. Finally, he was guided back into his heart.

> *Ego* – *'You need to keep working, it's what you are good at. You are needed to keep the business going.'*
>
> *Heart* – *'I feel lost. I want to be loved. Give up work and everything that you have achieved and go back to when you had nothing. That's the only way.'*
>
> *Ego* – *'How can you get to a place where you can balance work and home? How can you have the best of both worlds? If you give away your business this is giving away financial security and you need to bring up the family and have security.'*
>
> *Heart* – *'What's the point? What is important? It is the simple things. Living life together (with his wife and family).'*
>
> *Simon was very receptive to talking about his ego. He later reflected that identifying his ego was one of the most helpful aspects of therapy as it got to the core of his issues. By acknowledging this he was able to stop his ego dominating his life and move forward.*

It is important as therapists to remember that while it may sound easy to support our clients in just 'letting go of the ego,' it can be extremely difficult and challenging. We need to help to support them to come from a place of compassion. As therapists and clinicians, we have to recognise that our clients may have become best friends with their ego for a long time and it won't want to leave easily – it will put up a fight! We can highlight this to our clients and help them identify when their ego is trying to take charge. This has to be done gently and respectfully so as not to offend their ego, which will put up defences if it feels threatened or feels you are being judgemental in your manner. Our clients will make mistakes along the way, so with compassion we need to help them find ways to take care of themselves and accept that the journey will be bumpy; guiding them to learn to ride the waves of the storm rather than feel they are drowning in it, swimming in the tide of the waves rather than against them. Additional strategies and resources to teach clients on this journey are discussed throughout the book.

Brick walls or loving boundaries?

It is easy for clients to put up brick walls when they have experienced pain, suffering, and distress. This is a typical response that I am sure most of us can relate to. Brick walls become a defensive mechanism to try and prevent us from feeling hurt again. It can be easier to block out emotions and shut down our hearts than to experience pain. It is not unusual for clients who have undergone extreme trauma or abuse to dissociate completely from their emotions and/or physical bodies. This can be an effective survival strategy at the time and is what may have been necessary in order to get through the horrendous experiences. However, with time, those brick walls remain in place, firmly cemented, preventing the client from learning to experience positive affect or sensations. Thus, they live life in a numb state. If the client is continuing to live in a traumatic environment then obviously support is initially required to help them find a safer place to live free from the abuse. Once this is achieved, effective therapeutic interventions can be implemented to assist clients in being more present and process past trauma and attachment difficulties so that they no longer need to live life in a dissociative state. From a spiritual perspective, part of the healing work can include supporting clients in understanding what has happened in their life using HLP to bring down the brick walls safely and in their own time, so that they can replace these with loving boundaries. Teaching clients how to use protective loving boundaries (e.g. learning to speak up for themselves from a place of compassion but without relenting to others' perceived expectations or want of them) can allow them to start living a more authentic life. This enables them to open themselves up to receive, as well as give, unconditional love from their heart without becoming victims to abusive or destructive situations or people.

Case example of Simon's brick walls

Simon had put up brick walls to his marriage and family, his ego was ruling his life and telling him that he needed to keep being successful with his career in order to provide for his family. His wife had clearly told him that 'You can live without me but you can't live without your work.' Simon wasn't allowing himself to give or receive love because this made him feel insecure and vulnerable. When Simon started connecting to his heart and soul instead of his ego, he was learning what was really important to him – his family. In order to move forward and stop repeating past patterns of behaviour, Simon needed to start honouring his heart and soul and step away from his ego. This required him to take down the brick wall to his family. His fear of the unknown and belief that he could survive without being a workaholic was his biggest block, but he began to recognise the role his ego had in keeping his fear alive.

Drop the label or diagnosis

This may be a controversial area to discuss; whether we should be labelling and diagnosing clients. First, everyone is entitled to their opinion and it is not my aim to try and convert you to my way of thinking, but rather, to present a perspective for the benefits of avoiding labels as much as possible. There are some exceptions to this and if there are valid reasons why it would benefit the client to have a diagnosis in order for them to access necessary services educational, work or health support, then with their permission this can be advantageous. Unfortunately, we live in a world where labels and diagnoses are often heard more than the client's story. I personally try to avoid using labels or diagnoses unless under exceptional circumstances.

The ego loves labels and diagnoses because it gives clients an explanation or justification for why they feel the way they do, or why they behave in a certain way. Clients and their families may readily become dependent on labels and sometimes seek comfort in them. The difficulty is that they can keep the client feeling like a victim and powerless. Another difficulty with using labels and diagnoses is that they tend to stick – with superglue and they are surprisingly difficult to remove once they have been applied. Encouraging people to detach themselves from the label once it has been given is very tricky.

Case examples of dropping the label or diagnosis

Thomas was a gentleman in his early 70s who came to see me because he believed he had depression, severe depression. He wanted to get better but really struggled to shift from his diagnosis and would say 'But my GP told me it was SEVERE depression.' He was hooked on this diagnosis and constantly reminding himself about this understandably made him feel very negative. In actual fact it transpired that the GP had only made reference to 'severe' depression because he was supporting Thomas to get a reimbursement for his holiday insurance. While Thomas was experiencing some symptoms of low mood, he was not 'severely' depressed and we spent a number of sessions working at helping him to let go of his hook on this label – he had a very tight grip!

****

A couple came to see me because they were concerned their child had either Attention Deficit Hyperactivity Disorder (ADHD) or Oppositional Defiant Disorder (ODD). A family member had advised the couple to explore a diagnosis because of the difficulties they were experiencing with their child's behaviour at home. I explained before the initial appointment that I did not diagnose but thankfully they were keen to explore all options and gain a better understanding of the underlying issues. A detailed history revealed that their child, who was the eldest of three siblings, was feeling lonely, isolated, and had low self-esteem. The child was also struggling following his father changing jobs, which meant his father was not around as much. Formulating using an attachment perspective enabled the parents to empathise with their child and look at approaching their relationship in a different way, thus enabling their child to feel heard, loved and understood. They recognised that their child's behaviour was partly linked to the father's absence and started discussing how they could improve relationships at home. At the following session, both parents reported how they had started using a DDP approach, recognising a positive change in their child's behaviour, which was also acknowledged within the school.

I am sure we can all recall examples of clients who arrive having already diagnosed themselves, ranging from depressions and anxieties to personality disorders. Some may have formal diagnoses and can be prescribed heavy-duty medications. Whatever the situation, instead of using labels I still try to provide clients with an explanation of why they are struggling based on what has happened to them in their lives, using the BioPsychoSocioSpiritual model. It is frightening how even those clients who have formal diagnoses may have no understanding of the basis on which their diagnosis was made. Providing such formulations not only increases their understanding of their experiences, but also steers them away from labels, giving hope that there is potential to grow stronger and heal.

Letting go of the power of my ego

Let me be clear, I am on my spiritual journey, and my ego still appears regularly to keep me in check! By appearing at certain times, it helps remind me of how powerful and destructive it can be. When I become aware of the presence of my ego, I try to smile and thank it for this reminder and then I attempt to reconnect and centre on my heart and soul.

An example of a simple everyday challenge I can provide, which I am sure many of us can relate to, is when I received a rather patronising and derogative email from someone who had tangled me up in a situation where I was being used as a scapegoat and this was the second rather spiteful email I had received in a week. I was acutely aware that this person was deflecting a difficult issue they had created and, instead of facing up to their mistake, they were finding any opportunities to blame others, one of whom was myself. I then became conscious of feeling angry and the need to defend my position – my ego was being triggered. However, I didn't like what was happening to me. I could feel my ego really taking over and the resulting distress made me uncomfortable. With some patience and adopting a spiritual perspective I explored what this situation was trying to teach me; what could I learn from this experience in order to keep growing on my spiritual path? I asked myself 'How can I look at this situation with an open heart and with compassion?' This helped me move back into my heart and soul, to reconnect to my authentic self and as I did this, I became profoundly aware of feeling calmer in my body. I could easily have responded in a defensive manner and that was my initial reaction, but connecting with my heart and soul allowed me to proceed from a place of loving compassion, recognising that this person was feeling caught and trapped in their own mess and was probably really struggling in their own life. This challenge represented an opportunity for me to respond with self-belief, compassion, and integrity, while not taking on other people's judgements or criticisms.

Summary

- HLP teaches clients the impact of their ego on psychological distress and suffering.

- Teaching clients to have an awareness of their ego includes helping clients to understand how their egoic thinking creates fear, expectations, hooks and the victim role, all of which hold them back from moving into their heart and soul to make new choices and break free from repetitive themes in their lives.
- Clients can learn how to let go of hooks that are causing suffering. They can also be taught how to notice the different messages that their ego and heart and soul communicate to them.
- Clients can learn how to use loving boundaries rather than brick walls so that they can protect themselves in relationships by adopting a compassionate approach rather than shutting people off completely.
- HLP is not concerned with labelling or diagnosing clients. Instead, it aims to provide a formulation using a BioPsychoSocioSpiritual model of the difficulties clients have encountered, offering hope toward a deep healing by moving away from their ego and into their heart and soul to live a more authentic life.

4

Mindfulness

The source of now is here.

Rumi

This chapter focuses on mindfulness; mindfulness plays a significant role in HLP because it helps clients to become aware of when they are listening to their ego and provides different techniques for letting go of the ego and moving into their heart and soul. Used correctly, mindfulness can become a very powerful resource in life. I have worked with many clients, supervisees, and therapists, who have said they have learned some type of mindfulness, but when I explore this further I am often fascinated to discover that their understanding is somewhat limited to meditation rather than embracing mindfulness in all aspects of life. It is sometimes seen as an 'add-on' to help clients with a bit of resourcing for the occasional use, without really guiding them in how to live a mindful life and utilise it to its full capacity. This chapter begins by covering some of the research findings that support mindfulness in clinical work. A detailed script is then provided to enable you to teach your clients a thorough overview of mindfulness, as well as a separate mindful breathing exercise.

Mindfulness has become a buzzword, often thrown into conversations and mentioned on the radio, television programmes, social media, podcasts, etc., and there are numerous self-help and academic books available. The origins lie in Zen Buddhism as one of the stages or pathways leading to enlightenment. The benefits of mindfulness have been well researched over recent years and there is growing evidence in support of the application of mindfulness in many different clinical settings, in different client groups, with therapists, and for the general population as a whole (Ivtzan & Lomas, 2016). Jon Kabat-Zinn (1982) is acknowledged as the first person to apply mindfulness from Buddhist traditions to help patients with chronic pain. Since then, Mindfulness-Based Stress Reduction (MBSR) programmes have been proven to be a highly effective therapy for a broad range of physical health conditions for example chronic pain (Kabat-Zinn, Lipworth, Burncy, & Sellers, 1986) and MBCT has also been applied to other conditions of mental ill health (see Shapiro, de Sousa, & Jazaieri, 2016 for a review). The National Institute for

DOI: 10.4324/9781003613749-6

Health and Care Excellence (NICE, 2022) sites group mindfulness and meditation as one of the treatments of choice for mild depression. Mindfulness has been integrated into other forms of psychotherapy (Segal, Williams, & Teasdale, 2002) and is a core component in Dialectical Behaviour Therapy (Linehan, 1993) and Acceptance Commitment Therapy (Hayes et al., 2016). In the younger population, school-based mindfulness programmes have shown benefits for pupils in areas of academia and psychological well-being and resilience (Zenner, Herrnleben-Kuz, & Walach, 2014) as well as demonstrating a positive effect on cognitive performance, problem-solving skills, and attention (Zenner et al., 2014; Zoogman, Goldberg, Hoyt, & Miller, 2014). Mindfulness can be used from the age of six years old (Napoli, Krech, & Holley, 2005), and it has also been shown to increase children's ability to self-soothe, calm themselves, and be more present and less reactive (Abrams, 2008). In his book *The Body Keeps the Score*, Bessel Van der Kolk (2014) provided a compelling review of the research that shows how mindfulness has a positive impact on activating areas of the brain that are involved with emotional regulation, as well as many other physical benefits. Mindfulness practice has also been shown to be beneficial for clinicians in managing stress and promoting self-care (Irving, Dobkin, & Park, 2009; Shapiro & Carlson, 2009).

Mindfulness is not a religion; it is a way of being. Simply put, mindfulness is the practice of moving into one's awareness in the present moment. It is such an important part of HLP because if the client doesn't have awareness, they will not recognise when they are stuck in their challenges or egoic thinking and be able to follow the process of HLP.

Many clients who present to services with complex histories are dissociative to varying degrees. They have had to learn to dissociate as a way of coping and surviving terrible abuse and unthinkable distress in their lives. Mindfulness is the opposite of being dissociative. It is therefore essential that clients learn how to start engaging in the present moment and find new more effective ways of managing any discomfort. Some people may hold the view that learning to be mindful is the pre-requisite to finding inner happiness and peace in life, but I feel this oversimplifies the awful and traumatic experiences that clients have encountered. Learning mindfulness enables clients to engage with very powerful trauma therapies such as EMDR, trauma-focused Cognitive Behavioural Therapy and attachment work (such as DDP), which are often required to clear past traumatic memories. Teaching clients about mindfulness and making sure that they understand and apply this to their life can also be a very helpful clinical tool to demonstrate how ready they are to engage in further therapy. If a person is unable to even be present in the session with you or with aspects of their daily life, how can they be expected to engage at any level?

It is helpful to provide a thorough but uncomplicated overview of mindfulness to clients, which can get them started on this amazing journey and facilitate the further development of their mindfulness practice. I usually spend a session explaining mindfulness with most clients after completing a detailed history. Not only does it introduce them to the notion and benefits, but it will also help them to engage with the process of HLP, teach them how to embrace and manage difficulties moving forward and prepare them for more specific trauma work if required. I see my role as acting as a catalyst to introduce this topic and I do cover quite a lot of information during this session. It is a psycho-education session and my view is that once the client has a good understanding of mindfulness they can then start to implement this in their everyday life. I include how mindfulness can be used in an informal and formal way (Shapiro et al., 2016). I always check a client's understanding in subsequent sessions of how they are learning to implement mindfulness into their lives. Not everyone will need further support to grasp the concepts, sometimes the introduction is enough to get them going on this journey and they may choose to link into other support systems, courses or books to explore this further. Sometimes, however, clients do need additional support to really comprehend and implement the ideas, so we may spend several sessions working through this together.

Teaching mindfulness to your clients

Figure 4.1 illustrates what happens when we go into thinking mode. I describe this process as 'entering the Thought Bubble' and explain how negative thoughts cause distress using the following description and diagram.

Here is a diagram of a Thought Bubble and this is you here [point to the head shape below the Thought Bubble]. We are constantly bombarded with thoughts

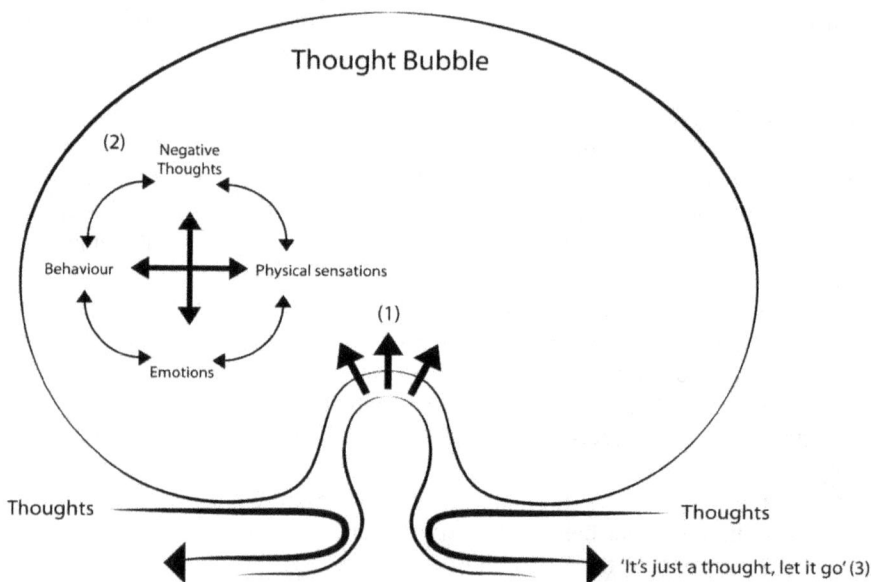

Figure 4.1 The Thought Bubble

in life. When a thought comes along and we engage with a thought we enter the Thought Bubble (1). When these are negative or unhelpful thoughts, they may set off a chain of thinking that is often about things that have happened in the PAST or what may happen in the FUTURE.

We often end up caught in a negative thought cycle (2). Negative thoughts (e.g. I am not in control, not good enough) effect our physical sensations, for example, we may notice our heart racing, butterflies in our stomach, sweating, tiredness, tearfulness, low motivation and energy, or getting hotter or colder in our body temperature. This can impact on our emotions; perhaps we start feeling sad, anxious, worried, or angry. Our behaviour then changes and we often want to avoid situations, seek reassurance from others, or carry out habits or certain behaviours which make us feel more in control. Unfortunately, while we think these behaviours are helping us, they are actually reinforcing negative thoughts. We then end up going around and around in a vicious negative cycle (2) where the thought gets stronger and more powerful, as do all the resulting physical sensations, emotions, and behaviours. Thinking about the PAST tends to lead to low mood or depression. Thinking about the FUTURE tends to create worries and anxiety.

Take a few moments to discuss with your client how this relates to their experiences so far in their lives. This helps to make it real to them.

When a thought comes along, we usually take it into our Thought Bubble (1). If it is a negative thought it may start small, but when we focus on this negative thought, the chain of thinking gets bigger and before we know it we have created a dramatic play or horror movie in our heads. In fact, we are the directors of our own horror movies. We quickly create a detailed, vivid, and complex scene of a play or story with lots of characters, either thinking about what has happened to us, or what may happen. We forget in the process that WE have created the play or movie because we are the directors. We could win Oscars for the plays we create! We are all very good at doing this, in fact, we have been doing this most of our lives. Research suggests that we spend approximately half our waking time in the Thought Bubble, but anecdotally I suspect it is much, much more than this. I used to be really good at this and I am sure you are too.

Usually at this point the client is very engaged and starts to recognise how they create their own horror movies. In fact, I have never had anyone who doesn't acknowledge their role. Discussing this in a non-judgemental way is essential for your client to be engaged and not feel embarrassed or ashamed.

Mindfulness is completely the opposite of being in the Thought Bubble. It is the practice of learning to become more aware in the PRESENT moment. It sounds simple, but in fact in reality it is incredibly difficult and challenging because we are so good at spending most of our time in the Thought Bubble.

Mindfulness is a journey in life. It isn't about 'getting to the end of the journey' or 'getting it.' Having that attitude or belief simply puts a block on the process, as we are giving ourselves an expectation of what we are trying to achieve and if we don't reach this, we judge or criticise ourselves. Instead, it is about learning to embrace the journey and the ride, the good parts and the tough parts, like learning to ride the crest of a wave and move in the direction of the water rather than trying to swim against the flow.

Mindfulness can be separated into two parts: an INFORMAL practice and FORMAL practice. Let me explain to you what I mean by this. The informal practice is starting to notice what is going on around you in the present moment using your physical senses. This means noticing what you can see, hear, smell, feel, touch and taste in the here and now. Let's just try that now. For a few moments I would like you to notice what you can hear in this present moment, just notice and then I will ask you to share your observations with me.

[Pause for a few minutes while also completing this exercise yourself]

Now can you tell me what sounds you noticed?

Spend a few minutes hearing back from your client about the sounds they heard. After they have finished, share the sounds you have heard too. Often people will notice the most obvious sounds, for example, the birds singing, doors opening or closing, background voices or traffic, but may not hear the more subtle noises, for example, the sound of their or your breath or the sound they make when they swallow. The more aware you become, the more you can bring their awareness to additional sounds that they hadn't first noticed.

Once you have both shared your experiences of sounds, complete the same exercise but this time ask your client to be aware of what they can see.

Now let's look around and notice what you can see. Just notice and then I will ask you to feed back to me in a few moments.

[Pause for a few minutes while also completing this exercise yourself]

Now can you tell me what you saw?

Again, first listen to your client's feedback before sharing what you noticed. People tend to notice the obvious, for example, the furniture or pictures in the room. I then bring their awareness slightly deeper by drawing their attention to the patterns or shadows of the furniture against the walls or floor, how the lights falls on different areas in the room, the tiny bubbles that may have formed in a glass of water, perhaps some indentations in the chairs from where someone sat previously.

Once you have shared your experiences of sight, complete the same exercise but this time ask your client to be aware of their physical sensations.

I am now going to ask you a few questions about what physical sensation you are noticing in this moment. If possible, try not to move or adjust yourself during this exercise. I would like you to just notice and then I will ask you to feedback your answers to me in a few moments.

Notice the weight of your body on the chair, is your body leaning in a particular way? Notice your feet, whether they are resting on the floor or is one foot balancing over one leg. Does this feel heavy or light, rough or smooth? Notice the contact points of your body on the chair and contact points between different body parts. Do certain parts of your body feel warm or cold?

Make this specific to the person you are with, so if they are sitting with their hands touching each other or resting on their lap or if they are wearing glasses, ask them to notice if they can feel these contact points.

Now can you tell me what physical sensations you noticed?

Spend a few minutes hearing back from your client. Usually by this stage your client has started to notice differences in body temperature, variations in their body in terms of heaviness or lightness, softness or roughness, contact points and so forth.

You can use the same exercise to illustrate what they notice when they eat, drink, and smell, depending on how much time you have available. This can be done at a further session if the person is finding it hard to grasp the concept and needs more practise. Sometimes I take clients for a mindful walk at a follow-up session if they are struggling to understand the true essence of informal mindfulness. I explain that we are going to walk in silence for several minutes noticing sounds, smells, and what we can see, hear, and feel physically. When we stop, I ask them for feedback on what they have noticed and then I also share what I have noticed. We continue doing this for the remainder of the walk, spending time in silence and then giving time for reflection and sharing. At the end of the walk I ask them what the experience was like. The majority of the time feedback is very positive because they are learning to notice so many things that they hadn't experienced before, and they also reflect that they feel calmer and more relaxed. This is because they have not been 'thinking' but instead they are 'being.'

The informal practice of mindfulness doesn't take any extra time in life. How you decide to get from one place to another or do activities during the day can either be done mindfully, or you can spend time in the Thought Bubble and be 'absent-minded' and not notice anything going on around you. For example, when you are in the car you may notice the road and traffic, but also notice the sky and patterns and shapes of the clouds, the scenery, or the music, or discussions on the radio. If you spend most of the journey in the Thought Bubble thinking about all the things you have just done, or need to do, you are likely to feel exhausted and stressed. Being mindful gives you a break from your thoughts and you are more likely to feel refreshed and uplifted and travel more safely.

The formal part of mindfulness is what I refer to as meditation and this does require you to put aside some time in the day, between five to 45 minutes depending on what you can manage. Meditation is not a religion and you do not have to have any specific belief system to meditate. It is nothing wackier than finding time to sit in a quiet place and notice what is going on WITHIN you – both physically and emotionally. When we start to go within, we may notice some tension or stress in our bodies, or feelings such as anxiety, anger or sadness. Most of the time we don't like these sensations or feelings and we push them away and try to get rid of them. The difficulty is that when we push the discomfort away, it is like putting a piece of coal on a fire – it actually keeps the fire going and makes the discomfort worse. This is because we are putting power into the discomfort and we become caught in a battle with it.

Mindfulness meditation takes the completely opposite approach. It encourages us to befriend what we are noticing within and welcome, embrace and greet the discomfort like an old friend, so that we can learn to sit and be comfortable with whatever arises. Emotions such as sadness, fear and anxiety are all normal healthy emotions, but over time we have learned to dislike them and be afraid of experiencing them. Befriending difficult sensations and feelings means there is no power struggle, and with time the discomfort dissolves away. This often takes a lot of practise and can be very challenging to do at first, but as we learn to be able to sit with whatever comes up or is going on within us, we are no longer afraid of embracing and being with the difficulty or discomfort. We let go of the fear of experiencing.

There are several important key concepts to consider in mindfulness. The first is AWARENESS. In essence, mindfulness is awareness. Practising both informal and formal mindfulness helps to increase our awareness. The more aware we become in life, the more we recognise when we are in the Thought Bubble and we can then step out of it by noticing what is going on in the present moment. Meditation is also a wonderful way of increasing our awareness and capacity to tolerate discomfort.

The second key concept is ACCEPTANCE. Mindfulness teaches us to accept whatever is happening around and within us. We learn to accept ourselves, our emotions and our feelings with loving kindness. We accept that on tricky days we may struggle to be more mindful and find ourselves spending more time in the Thought Bubble, but on other days it is less challenging. Life is a journey with ups and downs and it is not about getting it right. It is learning to experience whatever is in any given moment. Some days if I haven't slept well I may wake up and feel very tired. I could go into the Thought Bubble and create stories about how tired I am and worry about how I am going to get through the day because of my tiredness. Alternatively, I could notice my tiredness and accept it, allow it to be within me and embrace it. Doing this will probably mean I get through the day more easily, more peacefully and I will feel less tired than if I continued to focus on the discomfort, because I am not giving the tiredness any additional fuel from my thoughts.

The third concept is COMPASSION. It can be challenging to be compassionate to others but it is even harder to be compassionate to ourselves. This means treating and accepting all parts of ourselves with loving kindness and learning to find ways to nurture ourselves, including the parts of us that we find difficult to accept. Examples of nurturing ourselves might include finding time to meditate or do some hobbies or activities, saying something kind to ourselves, or acknowledging our achievements (big and small) during the day.

Finally, it is important to be NON-JUDGEMENTAL. Again, it is hard not to judge others but even harder not to judge ourselves. We are very good at being our own worst enemies and beating ourselves up using critical, blaming, judgemental thinking, which then makes us feel guilty and ashamed. When we do this it is as if we are stabbing ourselves repeatedly with a dagger or knife. We need to first become aware of when we do this and then learn to compassionately put down the weapon. Learning to forgive ourselves and others if we are judging ourselves or perceive we are being judged, can be an important part of this work. Starting to let go of what others think about us and trying not to live our lives by our perception of other people's judgements will help instead to embrace a life that is truer to you.

If we go back to the diagram of the Thought Bubble, you may recall that I said earlier that we are often bombarded by lots of thoughts in life. Mindfulness isn't about getting rid of thoughts or never being in the Thought Bubble – that is impossible. Some thoughts are really important, especially the positive thoughts that help us to function in life or can make us feel good about ourselves or our relationship to the world around us. What we learn to do is have a different and healthier relationship with our thoughts. Mindfulness can help us to learn to distinguish between negative unhelpful thoughts and the positive helpful ones. The negative thoughts only have POWER when we engage with them and take them into the Thought Bubble (1). If we don't do this, they are just thoughts. Mindfulness is recognising when the negative thoughts arrive and learning to let these thoughts move on past by just noticing them, rather than engaging with them. I like to think of a curvy arrow and say, 'It's just a thought let it go' (3), and then imagine the negative thought moving away from me. I may need to do that many times to start with, but this is far healthier than engaging with the thought and starting to create a horror movie in the Thought Bubble. Sometimes people like to visualise putting their thoughts on a cloud and watching it drift away, or putting it into a stream and watching it float away, or watching it move past them on a conveyor belt. It doesn't really matter, it is more important that you find something that works comfortably for you. The whole idea is to learn to accept that while thoughts are going to come during the day, we do not need to get angry or cross when this happens or to chastise ourselves. We just notice and learn to move the negative or distressing thoughts on by. If we notice that we have entered the Thought Bubble, we do exactly the same, first noticing and then letting the thought go, rather than enter into a debate about the thought or needing to justify its existence. We take a step back, and just compassionately let the thoughts move away from us.

Mindful breathing

The final part of the session on mindfulness is teaching clients how to use the breath as an effective and powerful way of learning to be mindful in the moment. It is also a gentle way of introducing the formal part of meditation into their lives.

The breath is always within us while we are alive. Learning to connect to the movement of the breath into and out of our bodies is an amazing and powerful way of bringing ourselves back into the moment. We can use mindful breathing wherever we are and whatever situation we find ourselves in, whether at home, work or school, or when we are out somewhere. It is probably one of the most beneficial resources I regularly use throughout the day. What I would now like to do is a mindful breathing guided meditation with you that lasts approximately six minutes. All you have to do is follow the instructions. Don't worry if your mind wanders, or if you notice thoughts start popping into your head. When you notice this, just bring your attention back to the movement of your breath into and out of your body. Part way through the meditation exercise I am going to ask you to start counting your breath; in for one, out for two, in for three, out for four, and we will continue to do this all the way to 20. When we reach 20 we will start with one again. You are not meant to hold your breath for these numbers, but instead just count the number of the breath to remind you of where you had got to in the process.

I then play a recording of mindfulness breathing which is available on YouTube ('Mindfulness Breathing' by Alexandra Dent) and I do this meditation alongside my client. I believe it is helpful to give clients a link to this meditation exercise so that they can practise in between sessions until they have grasped the essence themselves. If the client would prefer to hear your voice, you could read the mindful breathing script below, recording this on your client's phone during the session.

Exercise 3

Mindful breathing script

The first thing I would like you to do is to find somewhere quiet to sit for the next few minutes, get yourself into a really nice comfortable position sitting down, legs uncrossed, feet on the floor, rest your hands on your lap and if it feels comfortable close your eyes, or if you prefer, just settle yourself on a neutral gazing spot in front of you.
[Pause]
Then start to bring your awareness to the movement of the breath into and out of your body … notice how the air enters your nose into your lungs … and then back out from your lungs through your nose into the room again … Don't try to speed it up or slow it down, just allow it to be whatever it needs to be in this moment in time.
[Pause]
Allow the breath to anchor you in this moment.
[Pause]
Anytime those thoughts try and creep on in, just notice them and accept them and just allow them to pass on by … bringing your awareness back to the movement of the breath into and out of your body.

[Pause]

Sometimes it helps to think of the word CALM as you breathe in ... breathing in the calmness into the whole of your body ... and then think of the words LETTING GO as you breathe out ... breathing in the calmness and then letting go.

[Pause]

Just notice those thoughts as they try and come on in, don't get cross with them, just notice them and allow them to move on past, bringing your awareness back to the breath.

[Pause]

Breathing in the calmness and then letting go.

[Pause]

In a moment I would like you to start counting the breath, breathing in for the count of one ... out for the count of two ... in for the count of three ... out for the count of four, all the way to 20, and when you reach 20, start with one again. We are not trying to hold your breath for these numbers, instead just counting the number of breaths.

So let's start by letting go of any of the air in your lungs, just breathing that out, and with the next breath in, breathing in for one ... then out for two ... breathing in for three ... out for four, and continue this in your own time all the way to 20, and when you reach 20 just start with one again.

[Pause]

Just noticing any of those thoughts that try and come in, just notice and allow them to move on past.

[Longer pause]

And then wherever you are with the movement of the breath, just start bringing your awareness to how your body is sitting on the chair, your feet resting on the floor, your hands resting on your lap. Notice the temperature of the air on your skin ... start wiggling your fingers and your toes ... and in your own time start opening up your eyes bringing your awareness back into the room.

After you have completed the mindful breathing, it is very important to obtain feedback from your client about how they found the exercise, keeping the question as open as possible. Ask them:

What was that like for you?

Most clients will report feeling a sense of calmness and will often be surprised that they were not caught up in their thoughts. If so, that is great, congratulate them on managing to just keep up with the movement of their breath during this time. If clients struggle to keep their eyes closed then of course they can still do this with their eyes open. They may find it helpful to watch and follow you as you role-model the breathing. Sometimes clients fall asleep during this exercise! If this is the case, gently explain to them the importance of staying mindfully awake when completing the exercise during the day, by keeping their awareness on the movement of their breath. They may find it more helpful to keep their eyes open, to begin with, as this minimises the chances of them drifting into sleep.

I then use the following explanation with clients to illustrate how they can use mindful breathing during the night if they often wake up and struggle to get back to sleep:

> When we use mindful breathing throughout the day, the intention is to stay mindfully awake. However, if you are struggling with sleep: either dropping off to sleep or finding yourself waking up in the night and being plagued by thoughts, using mindful breathing at night time is a really effective way of bringing your awareness back to your breath and letting go of the thoughts. This is when I find it helpful to count the breath as it is focusing my attention on the breath rather than any thoughts. If you are doing this at night time, it is ok to have the intention of falling back to sleep. Sometimes it can happen very quickly, sometimes it takes a bit longer, but regardless, when you bring your awareness to your breath, you will be in a calmer state and you will find it easier to fall back into sleep.

For most of my clients I generally encourage them to practise the informal part of mindfulness along with mindful breathing for a few weeks and then review. If this works well then they may want to start building up a meditation practice very slowly using other guided meditation exercises. My clinical experience has been that if clients can start to feel comfortable with the concepts of informal mindfulness and are learning how to do this throughout their day in addition to practising mindful breathing, then they may be interested in exploring further meditation exercises in their own time. There are many different types of guided meditation exercises they can follow; I often recommend Mark Williams and Danny Penman's book, *Mindfulness: A Practical Guide to Finding Peace in a Frantic World* (2011), which comes with a CD of guided exercises (these are also available on YouTube).

The New Extended Light Stream is an additional meditation exercise available on YouTube ('The New Extended Light Stream' by Alexandra Dent) and the script is provided below if you wish to make your own recording. It incorporates:

- Mindful breathing.
- Light stream where clients are guided to imagine a healing light filling their body.

- Grounding techniques where clients imagine roots from their body, like roots from an oak tree entering the ground below.
- Protection, where clients imagine themselves surrounded by a protective bubble or shield that only lets positive thoughts and energy enter.

The light stream part of this meditation is a slightly different version of the light stream technique that has been widely used for many years as a highly effective resource in the preparation stages of EMDR (Shapiro, 2018). There are other meditation exercises on YouTube and other sources with similar ideas so encourage your clients to have a search and find ones that work best for them.

Exercise 4

The New Extended Light Stream meditation exercise

The first thing I would like you to do is to find a quiet place for the next 10 minutes where you will not be disturbed and get into a comfy position, either sitting on a chair or lying down, and if it feels comfortable close your eyes or if you prefer, just settle yourself on a neutral gazing spot in front of you.

[Pause]

Then start to bring your attention to your breath and notice the movement of air into and out of your body ... Don't try and speed it up or slow it down ... just accept it is what it is meant to be at this moment in time. Notice the movement of air entering your nose and into your lungs ... and then leaving your lungs ... back through your nose and out of your body. Sometimes it helps to think of the word CALM as you breathe in, ... breathing in the calm into the whole of your body ... and then think of the words LETTING GO as you breathe out ... breathing out all the stress and tension you may be holding onto inside.

[Pause]

Breathing in the calm and then letting go.

[Pause]

Now I want you to imagine a beautiful light stream above your head, as if someone is shining down a torch full of the most beautiful healing light. Ever so gently, I want you to imagine this healing light entering the top of your head and filling your head and face full of this beautiful healing light, filling every cell in your head and face full of this light, very calm and relaxed and letting go of any of the stress and tension, any of the worries that you might be holding on to, just imagine them all dissolving away and filling that space that is remaining with the healing light.

[Pause]

Once your head and face are full of the light, I want you to imagine that it is gently going to flow down your throat and neck and at your shoulders, I want you to imagine the light separating into two parts; one part flowing down your left arm and the other part flowing down your right arm. Imagine this healing light gently flowing down your arms, relaxing and soothing as it flows, flowing down to your elbows, down to your wrists and hands, and all the way to the tips of your fingers.

[Pause]

Then bringing your attention back to your shoulders, I want you to allow more of this healing light to gently flow down the front of your body and down your back, flowing down through your chest and your lungs and your heart, down through your spine and your ribs, gently flowing down through your stomach and your bowels, releasing the tension and stress and just filling that space with this beautiful healing light. Just notice the calmness and relaxation as it flows through your body.

[Pause]

At the top of your hips, I want you to again imagine the light separating into two parts; one part going down your left leg, the other part down your right leg. Allow this healing light to gently flow down your legs, down to your knees, down to your ankles and all the way to the tips of your toes, again letting go of any stress or tension you might be holding on to in these areas.

[Pause]

Now your whole body is full of this beautiful healing light. Just take a moment or two to notice the wonderful feeling inside your body, like the sunshine glowing, the warmth inside, and just enjoy the feelings it is creating with the healing light flowing around, making sure it reaches every part of your body. Any areas where there might be a slight blockage, give yourself permission to let go and allow the light to gently dissolve away the stress in that area.

[Pause]

Still keeping your eyes closed, I want you to imagine roots coming from the base of your feet, spreading deep, deep down into the earth below, spreading further and further down, making you feel very secure, very strong and grounded. Now I invite you to imagine your body is like the trunk of a wise old oak tree, full of this healing light, feeling very secure in the ground below.

I would like you to imagine that you are surrounded by a protective bubble, a very special bubble that only allows the positive thoughts and moments in life to enter. Any of the negativity or stress from the outside world just bounces off the edge of the bubble, sent back into the universe.

But the protective bubble surrounds you and allows the good positive, happy thoughts through. You may wish to fill the space between yourself and the edge of your protective bubble with more of the healing light, making you feel even stronger, even more secure.

[Pause]

Holding on to this beautiful image of you being this strong wise oak tree, full of the beautiful healing light shining within, with strong deep roots into the earth and completely surrounded by this very protective bubble, I want you to very gently in your own time, start wiggling your fingers and wiggling your toes, just slowly become aware of the surface that you are lying or sitting on, just start noticing ... and very gently when you are ready start opening up your eyes and coming back into the room, feeling much more relaxed, calm and very grounded.

Supporting clients who are highly dissociative

I would certainly not encourage clients who have a complex history to start formal meditation straight away. Learning to notice distress and discomfort in their bodies is likely to be overwhelming for such highly dissociative clients who may be very disconnected from their physical bodies and sensations. Instead I would encourage the informal mindfulness practice and see how they cope with that. Occasionally some clients really struggle even to engage in informal practice. This is an important clinical indicator and may highlight their level of dissociation and whether or not they are able to engage in more complex therapeutic work. For such clients they will need a lot more support and resource work to become more present. Jim Knipe's Back of the Head Scale (2015) is a valuable tool that can be used to teach clients an awareness of how present they are at any given time. This tool employs an imaginary line that runs from approximately one metre in front of their head (usually the distance from where their knees are when sitting upright) to the back of their head. The front of the line indicates being completely present and aware of everything going on around them in the present moment without the distraction of any thoughts. The back of the line indicates that your client is so lost in disturbing thoughts, images, feelings and sensations that they are completely absent-minded. You ask the client to indicate where they are currently on the line and if they are quite far back, encourage them to start using their informal mindfulness skills to move more forward and into the present moment. Sometimes completing a simple task such as throwing a cushion back and forth to your client can help them become more present in the room with you. The Back of the Head Scale is fantastic at helping clients to start increasing their awareness at any given stage in their day, as well as indicating how present they are in your sessions.

I cannot emphasise enough the importance of practising what you preach! If you are planning to use mindfulness with your clients, you must first experience it yourself, understand how it works, and be a good role-model to advocate the benefits. This means going far beyond reading a few books or attending a course. It requires you to practise mindfulness in your daily life. This in itself is often a challenge, but once it becomes a fundamental part of your day it is virtually impossible to imagine living without being mindful. Practise what you preach!

Further reading

There are many books available on mindfulness and it can be difficult to know where to start or what you can recommend to clients that portrays mindfulness in an accessible and uncomplicated way. Mark Williams and colleagues have written several informative and practical guidebooks on how to live mindfully and I would strongly encourage clinicians to read these, they are also a great resource to recommend to your clients. The Happy Buddha (2011, 2015, 2017) has also written several very helpful mindfulness books. Another lovely book is *Mindfulness: Plain and Simple* by Oli Doyle (2014), but if you are after a more in-depth and insightful read then I can highly recommend Beck and Smith's (1993) *Nothing Special: Living Zen*. A beautiful meditation book for children, which includes some spiritually based resources and meditations, is *The Wonder of Stillness* by Michelle Sorrell (2019).

Summary

- Mindfulness is 'awareness.' It is learning to connect to the present moment rather than being stuck in the Thought Bubble and thinking about the past or the future. While the concept of mindfulness is very simple, it can be very difficult to practise, because clients are so used to spending most of their time in the Thought Bubble.
- Mindfulness increases your client's capacity to contain their distress and difficulties. It has been well researched to show the benefits in many different client settings, groups, and ages, and within the general population.
- Mindfulness can be understood in both an informal way and a formal way. Teaching clients informal mindfulness helps them to connect to the present moment throughout the day using their senses and learning to let go of the thoughts that bombard them. This doesn't take any extra time, it simply requires your clients to notice and be present during the tasks that they are engaged with. All clients benefit from learning an informal approach to mindfulness.
- Formal mindfulness is teaching clients a process of meditation, taking some time in the day to connect with what is happening within themselves at both an emotional and physical level. This can be more challenging for some clients, especially those who are highly dissociative. For such clients, it is important that they first learn the informal process first before practising meditation.

- Key concepts of mindfulness include awareness, acceptance, compassion, and being non-judgemental.
- An essential part of HLP is to facilitate clients to become more mindful in their lives. Learning mindfulness will increase their awareness of challenges and therefore help them to follow the process of HLP.
- One way to demonstrate formal mindfulness is to teach clients various meditations including mindful breathing and the light stream meditation exercises. These can prove effective resources to utilise throughout the day, but also at nighttime if clients are struggling with sleep.
- It is essential to practise what you preach! If you are going to teach mindfulness, you must have experienced the process, understand it, and be a good advocate and role-model.

5

Learning to live a heart and soulful life

I will give you a new heart and put a new spirit in you; I will remove from you your heart of stone and give you a heart of flesh.

Ezekiel, 36:26

Having introduced the topic of the ego with your clients and shown them various techniques to recognise and then let go of their egoic thinking, including mindfulness, the next part of HLP is to teach your clients how they can connect with their heart and soul. In order to live through an open heart and soul rather than from the ego, clients have to learn to confront and accept their deepest fears. Part of this difficult challenge is learning to trust the process and take leaps of faith. This chapter provides guidance and exercises to support clients in forming a healthy relationship with their heart and soul. The idea of the 'Ful Trilogy' is also discussed, which includes mindfulness, heartfulness, and soulfulness, and Heartful and Soulful Meditation scripts are provided to assist with this process.

The heart has been a source of fascination and significance for thousands of years in Eastern and Western traditions, transcending its biological function. From a spiritual perspective it is considered to represent the source of unconditional love, compassion, courage, wisdom, the connection between the physical body with the spiritual self, higher realms, the Divine and a place where alchemy is possible. In the 4th century BCE Aristotle described the heart as 'The seat of the soul and the control of voluntary movement – in fact, of all nervous functions in general – are to be sought in the heart. The brain is of minor importance.' The *Book of the Dead* describes how the ancient Egyptians had a tradition of weighing the heart against the feather of the Ma'at (which symbolised truth). Only if the heart was lighter than the feather would one enter eternal paradise, known as the Field of Reeds. To achieve a light heart, one had to embrace gratitude for everything during one's life and not engage with negative thoughts or energies.

In the last century, research findings have provided scientific evidence to support the ideas of such ancient wisdom. In the 1960s and 1970s, John and Beatrice Lacey became recognised and respected as leading researchers when examining the interactions between the brain and heart from a psychophysiological perspective.

DOI: 10.4324/9781003613749-7

Neurocardiological research demonstrated how the heart has its own complex neural network with Armour (1991, 2008) suggesting that the heart has its own brain and nervous system containing as many as 40,000 neurones. The heart is believed to be composed of a complex network of ganglia, proteins, neurotransmitters, and support cells, referred to as the heart-brain. McCraty (2003, p. 3) described the heart as behaving like a 'sophisticated information encoding and processing centre that enables it to learn, remember, and make independent functional decisions that do not involve the cerebral cortex.' The heart has nerves from both the sympathetic and parasympathetic branches of the autonomic nervous system and will therefore be impacted by these as well as any emotions experienced. It is also able to function independently from the brain, having a neuronal network that is completely separate from the brain's descending sympathetic and parasympathetic control (Dispenza, 2017).

Often we identify the heart with its physical heart structure, but from a spiritual perspective it is generally believed to be located in the heart chakra. A chakra can be described as an energy centre in the body through which energy flows and it is believed that there are seven main chakras in the physical body that are thought to transform psychophysical energy into spiritual energy (Johari, 2000). The heart chakra is the fourth chakra in the body located at the exact centre of the chest. Yogic and Hindu traditions propose that it represents the place where the physical and spiritual come together and the source of unconditional love, or as O'Malley (2018) described, 'the centre of emotional empowerment.' McClintock (2015) reported the possibility of a deep healing of one's spiritual heart. When one connects with high vibrational emotions such as joy, bliss, love, compassion and gratitude, it enables one to move from a place of selfishness to selflessness (Dispenza, 2017).

In addition to the seven main chakras in the physical body, some believe there are other chakras both above and below the physical body. O'Malley provided a detailed description of each of these and what he believes is their corresponding functions; for example, suggesting that the ninth chakra (transcendental chakra) is the connection of the soul to the Divine Source. Wilber (2000) described communications from the soul as 'whispers of the soul,' believing that messages represent opportunities to connect with the higher self and facilitate healing. This can be a very personal experience, perhaps described as an awareness of a presence within that is connected to a higher source or a 'knowing.' Different forms of 'knowing' or intuition were described by Braud and Anderson (2002) ranging from visual, auditory, kinaesthetic, proprioceptive, and direct knowing, which can be developed through one's own personal spiritual practice, including meditation and training. I have noticed that the more I embrace and honour my soul dharma, my 'knowings/ intuition' have strengthened and developed, guiding me in all areas of my life including my work with clients.

Teaching clients to live life through the heart and soul ultimately means assisting them with relinquishing their ego, expectations, desires, ambitions, and needs. When clients can move into their heart and soul and start listening to what their heart and soul is trying to communicate with them, they realise that they have all the answers within themselves to start living a more authentic life. I believe that learning to connect with my soul has helped me to connect with my higher self and the Divine, supporting me on my spiritual path both personally and clinically.

Benefits of connecting with the heart and soul

Technology has demonstrated the benefits of living a heartful life. Heartmath (www.heartmath.com) is a biofeedback system founded by Doc Childre in 1991 to bridge the intuitive connection between heart and mind, enabling self-regulation of emotions and behaviours. Heartmath's aim is to help individuals to connect with their hearts to improve human interactions and create a more compassionate world. Their research measures heart rate coherence; the pattern of heart rate variability (HRV, the variation in time between heartbeats) that occurs when the heart, mind, and emotions synchronise into an ordered and harmonious rhythm. This coherence can be achieved by connecting to high-frequency emotions such as joy, bliss, love, and grace, while breathing slowly and rhythmically, thus enabling one to open up and deepen the relationship with one's heart (Dispenza, 2017). Childre and McCraty (2002) and Dispenza (2017) reported how individuals felt a deep connection with the creator during times of optimal cardiac activity. Research findings continue to grow in this area, showing a decrease in stress and improvement in resilience when in heart coherence which enables individuals to link into their natural intuition, higher guidance, wisdom and the quantum field thus facilitating the ability to make more healthy choices in their lives.

The heart has also been shown to produce the highest emissions of electromagnetic energy from the body which can be felt by others, regardless of whether touch is involved (McCraty et al., 1998). Dispenza believes that the electromagnetic fields emitted from the human body and heart are able to interact with external fields in the environment, including the Earth's geomagnetic field and other energy fields. When these fields come into resonance with each other, healing, transformation, and enhanced states of consciousness is possible (Dispenza, 2017). He also discovered that when an individual is in heart coherence and balance, the magnetic field within and beyond themselves has an impact on the heart of other individuals, irrespective of whether they are in different locations. Dispenza's findings along with data from the HeartMath Global Coherence Initiative propose an invisible field that enables information to be transmitted to all living things including collective human consciousness. This energy field has the ability to influence people's behaviours, thoughts, emotions, and conscious and unconscious thoughts which, of course, can be both positive or negative depending on the emotional or cognitive frequency to which a person is connecting. This idea may explain why it is possible to achieve a strong therapeutic relationship and spiritual resonance between therapist and client when working online, if, of course, the therapist is taking responsibility for their own heart coherence and energetic state. The idea of an electromagnetic invisible field also led to global meditations being organised, initiated by Project Coherence in 2015, where over 6,000 individuals connected online during heartful Meditations with the intention of manifesting a more peaceful world. Since then, this has resulted in a significant increase in organised group Heartful Meditations, especially during times of conflict or trauma.

When using HLP it is important to ask yourself as a therapist whether you know how to connect with your own heart and soul. Are you a good role model for your clients to help support them through this process? When Siegel (2013) investigated spiritual resonance within therapists, she found that some reported connecting with their clients 'heart-to-heart.' One therapist described this spiritual resonance as creating a heart loop, where he observed light shining from his heart to his client's heart, facilitating the release of energy blocks. Other therapists recognised themselves as a vessel or channel for spiritual resonance and some reported awareness of a soul consciousness within their clients, where they were starting to awaken to their spirituality and become more engaged in spiritual activities beyond the therapeutic work. Therapists also noticed how their client's hearts were opening up more generally in their lives to make healthier changes, sometimes removing themselves from activities or people that were no longer serving a healthy purpose to them. HLP aims to assist clients to form a stronger connection with their heart and soul. A case example of this is given in Chapter 10 with Marie, where HLP-informed EMDR helped her to start connecting and understanding the messages from her heart instead of her ego, with the realisation during EMDR processing that it was her heart that was keeping her alive.

Teaching your clients strategies to connect with their heart and soul

The next part of this chapter provides a range of practical exercises and meditations that you can use with your clients to help them connect to their heart and soul. For many clients this will feel rather new, because they are so used to living in their own 'Thought Bubble' and listening to their ego, but as they practise these strategies they will start to feel more comfortable in themselves, recognise the benefits and actually want to make changes in their life which are more in keeping with their heart and soul.

Exercise 5

Bringing awareness into the heart and soul

When a client is struggling to make an important decision that is causing them discomfort or suffering, I use this exercise to teach them to start moving away from their ego and connect with their heart and soul. It is different to Exercise 2 (in Chapter 3) where a conversation can be had between the ego and heart, because it encourages clients to stay within their heart and soul and consider different options for a situation as they rest there. When clients learn to bring their awareness to these areas they can then bring to mind different scenarios and observe how their body or guidance from their hearts change, either physically or emotionally, which can then assist them in decision-making. For simplicity, I refer to the heart with clients as the place in their body that is their source of unconditional love, compassion, authenticity and their emotional centre. If in doubt, or if this does not resonate with your client, ask them what their heart represents to them, making sure this is not coming from their ego. When a client is open to the concept of a soul, this may represent the place where they feel connected to their higher self or presence, their intuition or just a 'knowing.' For each person it may represent something slightly different so try to be open to what is true to your client rather than impose your own views.

The instructions for this exercise are as follows:

What I would like you to do is bring your awareness into your heart area. The heart area may represent your source of unconditional love, compassion and your truth. Just rest there for a moment and start to really feel connected to this space.

[Pause]

When you are ready I would like you to bring to mind the first scenario that you were considering.

[Pause]

Now move your awareness into your heart area and just settle there for a moment.

[Pause]

Notice any changes in your body or feelings as you are considering this scenario from your heart.

[Pause]

Now what I would like you to do is bring to mind the other scenario that you were considering.

[Pause]

Now move your awareness into your heart area and just settle there again for a moment.

[Pause]

Notice any changes in your body or feelings as you are considering this alternative option.

[Pause]

What did you notice happen when you considered either option?

Allow your client time to feedback to you what they noticed in their body and emotions as they considered both scenarios from their heart and ask them to reflect on what the exercise was like for them.

Adding the soul

If your client is open to the concept of a soul, I would add this to the exercise as follows:

What I would like you to do is bring your awareness into your heart and soul area. The heart area may represent your source of unconditional love, compassion and your truth. Your soul area may be that place in you that is your intuitive self, your connection with your higher self or just a knowing. Just rest there for a moment and start to feel really connected to this space.

[Pause]

When you are ready I would like you to bring up the first scenario that you were considering.

[Pause]

Now move your awareness into your heart and soul areas and just settle there for a moment.

[Pause]

Notice any changes in your body or feelings as you are considering this option.

[Pause]

Now what I would like you to do is bring to awareness the other scenario that you were considering.

[Pause]

Now move your awareness into your heart and soul areas and just settle there again for a moment.

[Pause]

Notice any changes in your body or feelings as you are considering this alternative option.

[Pause]

What did you notice happen when you considered either option?

Allow your client time to feedback what they noticed in their bodies and emotions as they considered both scenarios and ask them to reflect on what that exercise was like for them. You can of course just do this for the soul area if your client wishes – remember to ask them what they would prefer.

Case example of Arjun connecting to his heart and soul

Arjun was briefly discussed in Chapter 2. We had a session after his family holiday and he was still struggling with his relationship with his wife.

He discussed various stressful situations that had happened during his holiday, including how his wife was asking him at the most inconvenient times whether their marriage was okay. He recognised that his ego was telling him that he couldn't leave her: what would happen to the children, how would he manage financially, how would his wife manage without him, what would happen if he grew old on his own? I asked Arjun to connect with his heart and soul and I gave him a few moments to settle there. I then asked him to bring up the scenario of staying with his wife and to notice in his heart and soul what was happening as he considered this option. After a while I asked him to bring up the other scenario of being on his own, connect with his heart and soul and notice what happened as he considered this alternative option. In his feedback, Arjun recognised his body tensing up at the thought of staying in his marriage with his wife, especially in his shoulders. As he moved to the other scenario he said he noticed a sense of relief and release. He could visualise himself being happy even when he was older and enjoying spending time with his children.

This proved to be a very powerful exercise for Arjun. His heart and soul knew what was right, it was his ego that was causing the blocks. The heart and soul holds the answers, if only we can show clients how to listen, acknowledge, and trust their guidance.

Exercise 6

Enriching versus draining activities

This exercise is in the resource section at the end of the book and is designed to help your client identify which activities in their life enrich or drain them at a heart and soul level. On the left-hand side of the table, clients are asked to identify enriching activities that make them feel good or alive, make their heart and soul sing for joy, make them feel self-compassionate or self-loving. This can include activities they are currently involved with, as well as those that they would like to start doing. On the right-hand side of the table, clients are asked to identify draining activities that they are currently involved with that make them feel exhausted, overwhelmed, and depleted.

It is beneficial if clients can be quite specific about each activity, so instead of just saying 'work' or 'children,' they are asked to reflect on whether there is anything in particular that is either enriching or draining; for example, attending meetings at work, commuting, responding to the numerous emails, asking the kids to come off their gadgets at bedtime, tidying up after the family, and so forth. Once they have identified key enriching and draining activities they are asked to rate how often they engage with these activities ranging from very often (daily) to rarely (once a month or less).

Clients are then asked to observe what they have put in the table and notice what stands out to them. Is their life balanced between enriching and draining activities, or have they filled their life with more enriching activities or draining activities? If they are out of balance, what needs to change to balance this out? Encourage your clients to think about how they could increase enriching activities so that they start to feel stronger and more joyful at a heart and soul level. Try to encourage clients to stay connected with their heart and soul as they do this exercise rather than slipping into their ego.

Exercise 7

Enriching versus draining people

This exercise is also in the resource section and is similar to Exercise 6 but this time it is identifying which people in your client's life enrich or drain them. On the left-hand side of the table, clients are asked to identify people who make them feel good or alive, make their heart and soul sing for joy, make them feel self-compassionate or self-loving. On the right-hand side of the table, clients are asked to identify people that drain them and make them feel exhausted, overwhelmed and depleted.

Once they have identified key enriching and draining people, they are asked to rate how often they have involvement with these people in their lives. Again, encourage your clients to be quite specific with this task, for example, when they go out with friends, are there certain individuals that make them feel alive and happy, or bored! At work, are there specific individuals who affect how they feel and do these individuals have the same impact on others in the workplace, or is it just specific to them? When with certain members of the family, do they feel their energy being drained or do they feel nourished and loved?

Having identified specific people, clients are then asked to observe what they have put in the table and notice what stands out to them. Is their life balanced between enriching and draining people or have they filled their life with more enriching or draining people? Are there more draining people, and if so what needs to change to balance this out? Encourage your clients to think about how they could increase being around people who make them feel more positive so that they can start to feel stronger and more joyful at a heart and soul level. Try to encourage clients to stay connected with their heart and soul as you do this exercise, rather than slipping into their ego.

Teaching your clients these exercises will help them become aware of whether their life is full of draining activities and people, full of enriching activities and people or whether they are more in balance. Understandably it may not be possible to eliminate some of the draining activities and people due to circumstances or requirements with work, family etc. However, the more aware they become, the more your clients can start noticing the impact of situations and people on their life and choices they make. This gives clients the option of learning how to manage such draining situations or people, perhaps by implementing resources and coping strategies or loving boundaries, and at least aim for a more balanced lifestyle in order to minimise the impact of anything that is draining. It is worth encouraging your clients to repeat these exercises regularly because situations will change in their life, so it helps to keep them self-aware so that they can act upon this knowledge rather than react.

Exercise 8

Positive referencing beliefs

This exercise is also found in the resource section. It is designed to help your clients to start having more helpful positive beliefs about themselves, especially if they have been caught in the victim role for a long time and perceive themselves in a very destructive or self-defective way. Negative thinking can easily spiral out of control and this will impact on a client's physical sensations, emotions, and behaviour. One way to try and tackle this is to ask your client to make a list of some positive self-referencing beliefs. If they struggle to think of many, then you can ask them how their close friends or family would describe them as a person and ask them what qualities others see in them. Once your client has come up with some ideas, ask them to write these down and say them regularly throughout the day, from the moment they wake up. This can help to balance out their negative thinking and with time can even cancel out the negative thoughts. They may also find it beneficial to put some positive referencing beliefs on sticky notes around the house to remind them to think positively about themselves.

Exercise 9

Positive affirmations

This exercise, described in the resource section is based on the belief:
What we think or believe, we manifest.

In other words, if your client believes everything is going to fail and nothing good will happen in their life, then this is more likely to be the outcome.

Holding on to positive affirmations not only improves your client's outlook and makes them feel more empowered, but also helps manifest what they are hoping for. Ask your client to construct a positive affirmation, examples of which are provided in this exercise and suggest that they write the affirmation down 10 times in the evening and say this out loud in the morning. Ask them to repeat for 10 days or as long as required. If during this time another situation arises and they would feel it beneficial to change their positive affirmation then by all means recommend that they do this. The key is to have a positive affirmation that fits the situation or challenge they are going through and helps to reinforce a positive outcome that they can manifest.

Your client needs to be realistic and not too specific when they write their affirmations. For example, if they put 'I am going to win the lottery,' then this may not happen! However, an alternative and more realistic affirmation could be 'all my financial and material needs are met.' This is much more likely to be manifested.

The Ful Trilogy

As my passion for mindfulness and my ability to meditate has developed over the years, I could not help but notice the whispers of my soul. Depending on what type of teaching is offered, some mindfulness teachings do not openly recognise the concept of a soul, perhaps referring to this presence as a consciousness in the here and now. While I discussed this with some mindfulness teachers, I was not actively encouraged to explore this, instead being guided to focus on the here and now. However, my awareness of my soul was so powerful that I could not ignore its existence. I believe my soul communicates to me at a profound level from both a physical feeling and an emotional sense. By starting to listen to my soul I have learned to make many changes in my life and I feel my soul has strengthened

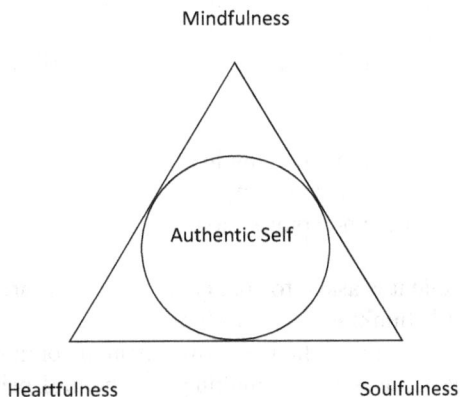

Figure 5.1 The Ful Trilogy

through this process. Listening to my soul has been a huge part of my spiritual journey and has ultimately led me to introduce spirituality into my clinical work as well as all other aspects of my life. If I hadn't listened to my soul, this book would never have been written!

Learning to live an authentic life often requires us to be mindful, heartful and/or soulful as illustrated in Figure 5.1. I don't want anyone to suggest that what I am saying is that if you don't recognise or acknowledge the presence of a soul then you cannot be authentic because this is not true, authenticity comes from living a heart led life. For some, acknowledging the presence of their soul will be very powerful and just adds another dimension to work with in the process of healing and becoming authentic.

The process of being heartful and soulful is very similar to being mindful. One could argue that mindfulness incorporates heartfulness and isn't a separate experience. The reason why I have called it the Ful Trilogy is that HLP requires your clients to really move specifically into their heart rather than anywhere else in their body and then start to notice what feels right when they rest in this place. Soulfulness does the same – some clients may not comprehend or connect with the presence of a soul and that is absolutely fine; honour what is right to them.

In addition to mindful breathing, your clients may find it helpful to use a Heartful and Soulful Meditation (both available on my YouTube channel; 'Heartful Meditation' by Alexandra Dent; 'Soulful Meditation' by Alexandra Dent) so that they can start to experience what it is like when connecting with their heart and soul. The more aware they become, the easier they will find it to move away from their ego and start utilising the strategies of HLP discussed in the following chapters. A Heartful and Soulful Meditation script is provided below to use with your clients so that you can make your own recording if your clients prefer to hear your voice.

Heartful Meditation

The Heartful Meditation exercise is similar to the Loving Kindness Meditation (The Happy Buddha, 2015) or the Befriending Meditation (Williams & Penman, 2011). In each of these there are five optional stages where a few phrases are held in mind while being connected to the heart area (as described in Exercise 5). The phrases in Heartful Meditation are:

May I be open to giving and receiving love,
May I be free from suffering and pain,
May I live a life of grace and compassion.

In the first stage, the client is asked to connect to their heart area and bring to mind the above phrases while thinking of themselves. The second is to repeat the phrases while thinking of a close person who has shown them unconditional love. The third stage is to repeat the phrases while thinking of a neutral person (someone they may see at the supermarket or when out walking, but with whom they do not have any personal connection with) and the fourth stage is to repeat the phrases while thinking of someone who has caused them discomfort or suffering. Finally, the phrases are repeated and may be extended as far as the mind will allow to include all living beings, creatures, and life on the planet and universe. At the beginning, some clients will only be able to manage to complete the first stage and this is absolutely fine. They mustn't feel any pressure to push themselves further than they feel able to at any given point or it defeats the purpose of the exercise. With time, they may be able to extend these wishes to other people. By doing this, it allows their heart to open up so that they can learn to give as well as receive unconditional love.

Exercise 10

Heartful Meditation script

The first thing I would like you to do is to find somewhere quiet to sit for the next few minutes, get yourself into a really nice comfortable position sitting down, legs uncrossed, feet on the floor, rest your hands on your lap and if it feels comfortable close your eyes or if you prefer, just settle yourself on a neutral gazing spot in front of you.

[Pause]

Then start to bring your awareness to the movement of the breath into and out of your body ... notice how the air enters your nose into your lungs ... and then back out from your lungs through your nose into the room again ... Don't try to speed it up or slow it down, just allow it to be whatever it needs to be in this moment in time.

[Pause]

Allow the breath to anchor you in this moment.

[Pause]

Any time those thoughts try and creep on in, just notice them and accept them and just allow them to pass on by ... bringing your awareness back to the movement of the breath into and out of your body.

[Pause]

When you are ready, bring your awareness into your heart area and just rest there for a few moments. The heart area may represent your source of unconditional love, compassion and your truth. Notice whether there is any discomfort or tension or perhaps a sense of calmness and peace. Just allow whatever comes up to come up without censure or judgement, using your breath to breathe into your heart area.

[Pause]

Connecting with your heart area, bring up the phrases:

May I be open to giving and receiving love,
May I be free from suffering and pain,
May I live a life of grace and compassion.

Imagine each of these phrases gently dropping into your heart area. Be aware of whether there is any resistance or tension as you do this and using your breath, see whether you can embrace these sensations with loving kindness and acceptance.

[Pause]

Remaining connected to your heart area, if you so choose, bring to mind a close friend or family member who has shown you unconditional love in your life. Notice any sensations that arise and just accept these as true to you in this moment, without censure or judgement.

[Pause]

When you are ready and feel connected to this person, offer them the following phrases:

May you be open to giving and receiving love,
May you be free from suffering and pain,
May you live a life of grace and compassion.

Imagine each of these phrases gently dropping into your heart area. Be aware of whether there is any resistance or tension as you do this and using your breath, see whether you can embrace these sensations with loving kindness and acceptance.

[Pause]

Still connected to your heart area, and if you so choose, bring to mind someone who is neutral in your life. This may be someone you notice when travelling to work, in the supermarket, or when you are out walking. Just like you, they too may wish for a calm life, free from suffering and pain. Notice any sensations that arise as you bring this person to mind and just accept these as true to you in this moment, without censure or judgement.

[Pause]

When you are ready and feel connected to this person, offer them the following phrases:

May you be open to giving and receiving love,
May you be free from suffering and pain,
May you live a life of grace and compassion.

Imagine each of these phrases gently dropping into your heart area. Again, just be aware of whether there is any resistance or tension as you do this and using your breath, see whether you can embrace these sensations with loving kindness and acceptance.

[Pause]

Remaining connected to your heart area, the next part is to bring to mind someone who has upset you or caused suffering or discomfort to you. Just like you, they too may wish for a calm life, free from suffering and pain. Notice any sensations that arise as you bring this person to mind and just accept these as true to you in this moment, without censure or judgement. If this is too difficult, then just bring your awareness back to your breath.

[Pause]

If you feel able to continue, when you are ready and feel connected to this person, offer them the following phrases:

May you be open to giving and receiving love,
May you be free from suffering and pain,
May you live a life of grace and compassion.

Imagine each of these phrases gently dropping into your heart area. Just be aware of whether there is any resistance or tension as you do this and using your breath, see whether you can embrace these sensations with loving kindness and acceptance.

[Pause]

Finally, connecting to your heart area, and if you so choose, we are going to extend this Heartful Meditation as far as you feel able, to everyone in your street, home town, county, country, the entire planet and universe. This can include all living creatures. Just like you, they too may wish for a calm life, free from suffering and pain. Notice any sensations that arise as you extend your mind as far as you feel able and just accept these as true to you in this moment, without censure or judgement.

[Pause]

When you are ready and feel connected to every living being and creature that you wish to include, offer them the following phrases:

May you be open to giving and receiving love,
May you be free from suffering and pain,
May you live a life of grace and compassion.

Imagine each of these phrases gently dropping into your heart area. Again, just be aware of whether there is any resistance or tension as you do this and using your breath see whether you can embrace these sensations with loving kindness and acceptance.

[Pause]

Now for a few minutes, bring your awareness back to your breath and the movement of the breath into and out of your body.

[Pause]

And then wherever you are with the movement of the breath, just start bringing your awareness to how your body is sitting on the chair, your feet resting on the floor, your hands resting on your lap. Notice the temperature of the air on your skin ... start wiggling your fingers and your toes ... and in your own time start opening up your eyes, bringing your awareness back into the room.

Soulful Meditation

The Soulful Meditation is similar to the Heartful Meditation but this time connecting at a soul level. This may be a particular place in the body, all over, or just an awareness of the presence of the higher sense, a sense of 'knowing' or 'intuition' at a soul level. It is important not to force anything to happen, just connect with whatever comes up at a soul level. This can be further extended to connecting to a higher source, whether it is the Divine Source, God, one's own personal team of guides, teachers, helpers, and angels. It is important to make sure the intention is set to only ask for support and guidance that comes from a loving, positive source that is for the highest good.

As with the Heartful Meditation, there are five optional stages and when connecting to the soul the following phrases are held in mind before dropping them into the soul:

May I live an authentic, heart and soulful life,
May I live a life of ease and grace,
May I be the best version of myself that I can be.

Exercise 11

Soulful Meditation script

The first thing I would like you to do is to find somewhere quiet to sit for the next few minutes, get yourself into a really nice comfortable position sitting down, legs uncrossed, feet on the floor, rest your hands on your lap and if it feels comfortable close your eyes or if you prefer, just settle yourself on a neutral gazing spot in front of you.

[Pause]

Then start to bring your awareness to the movement of the breath into and out of your body ... notice how the air enters your nose into your lungs ... and then back out from your lungs through your nose into the room again ... Don't try to speed it up or slow it down, just allow it to be whatever it needs to be in this moment in time.

[Pause]

Allow the breath to anchor you in this moment.

[Pause]

Anytime those thoughts try and creep on in, just notice them and accept them and just allow them to pass on by … bringing your awareness back to the movement of the breath into and out of your body.

[Pause]

When you are ready, bring your awareness to where you feel you connect with your soul and just rest there for a few moments. This may be a particular place in your body, all over or you may just be aware of the presence of your higher sense, a sense of 'knowing' or 'intuition' at a soul level. Don't try to force anything to happen, just allow yourself to connect with whatever comes up, holding in mind yourself at a soul level. You may then choose at a soul level to connect to a higher source whether it is the Divine Source, God, or your own personal team of guides, teachers, helpers and angels. Make sure you set the intention to only ask for support and guidance that comes from a loving, positive source which is for your highest good. Notice whether there is any discomfort or tension or perhaps a sense of calmness and peace. Just allow whatever to come up to come up without censure or judgement, using your breath to breathe into your soul.

[Pause]

Connecting with your soul, bring up the phrases:

May I live an authentic, heart and soulful life,
May I live a life of ease and grace,
May I be the best version of myself that I can be.

Imagine each of these phrases gently dropping into your soul. Be aware of whether there is any resistance or tension as you do this and using your breath, see whether you can embrace these sensations with loving kindness and acceptance.

[Pause]

Remaining connected to your soul, if you so choose, bring to mind a close friend or family member who has shown you unconditional love in your life. Notice any sensations that arise and just accept these as true to you in this moment, without censure or judgement.

[Pause]

When you are ready and feel connected to this person, offer them the following phrases:

May you live an authentic, heart and soulful life,
May you live a life of ease and grace,

May you be the best version of yourself that you can be.

Imagine each of these phrases gently dropping into your soul. Be aware of whether there is any resistance or tension as you do this and using your breath see whether you can embrace these sensations with loving kindness and acceptance.
   [Pause]
   Still connected to your soul, and if you so choose, bring to mind someone who is neutral in your life. This may be someone you notice when travelling to work, in the supermarket or when you are out walking. Just like you, they too may wish for a calm life, free from suffering and pain. Notice any sensations that arise as you bring this person to mind and just accept these as true to you in this moment, without censure or judgement.
   [Pause]
   When you are ready and feel connected to this person, offer them the following phrases:

May you live an authentic, heart and soulful life,
May you live a life of ease and grace,
May you be the best version of yourself that you can be.

Imagine each of these phrases gently dropping into your soul. Again, just be aware of whether there is any resistance or tension as you do this and using your breath, see whether you can embrace these sensations with loving kindness and acceptance.
   [Pause]
   Remaining connected to your soul, the next part is to bring to mind someone who has upset you or caused suffering or discomfort to you. Just like you, they too may wish for a calm life, free from suffering and pain. Notice any sensations that arise as you bring this person to mind and just accept these as true to you in this moment, without censure or judgement. If this is too difficult, then just bring your awareness back to your breath.
   [Pause]
   If you feel able to continue, when you are ready and feel connected to this person, offer them the following phrases:

May you live an authentic, heart and soulful life,
May you live a life of ease and grace,
May you be the best version of yourself that you can be.

Imagine each of these phrases gently dropping into your soul. Just be aware of whether there is any resistance or tension as you do this and using your breath, see whether you can embrace these sensations with loving kindness and acceptance.

[Pause]

Finally, connecting to your soul, and if you so choose, we are going to extend this Soulful Meditation as far as you feel able, to everyone in your street, home town, county, country, the entire planet, universe and creation. This can include all living creatures. Just like you, they too may wish for a calm life, free from suffering and pain. Notice any sensations that arise as you extend your mind as far as you feel able and just accept these as true to you in this moment, without censure or judgement.

[Pause]

When you are ready and feel connected to every living creature that you wish to include, offer them the following phrases:

May you live an authentic, heart and soulful life,
May you live a life of ease and grace,
May you be the best version of yourself that you can be.

Imagine each of these phrases gently dropping into your soul. Again, just be aware of whether there is any resistance or tension as you do this and using your breath, see whether you can embrace these sensations with loving kindness and acceptance.

[Pause]

Now for a few minutes, bring your awareness back to your breath and the movement of the breath into and out of your body.

[Pause]

And then wherever you are with the movement of the breath, just start bringing your awareness to how your body is sitting on the chair, your feet resting on the floor, your hands resting on your lap. Notice the temperature of the air on your skin ... start wiggling your fingers and your toes ... and in your own time start opening up your eyes, bringing your awareness back into the room.

Happiness versus grace

A key point to remind clients is that embracing a spiritual journey is an individual experience. It is important for our clients to be clear about what their intention is from the outset. Do they want to have a deeper understanding of their life so far and the challenges they have experienced? Many people spend their lives striving or searching for happiness and view this as the answer to their difficulties. There are several books written to guide people in search of happiness, often by living a mindful life. However, Villoldo (2005) said that happiness is fleeting and casual and that grace instead is more transformative. Grace enables us to be fully ani-mated or awakened in life. He said that 'in grace, you're free to be like the "lilies of the field" who need nothing, or those who "walk in the shadow of death and fear no evil," you just are.' Villoldo also suggested that grace is achieved when the soul is completely healed from all past life wounds with the gained insight and wisdom from what caused the soul trauma. To me this represents authenticity, where a per-son lives a life of values and morals that are true to them and are based on pure unconditional love, rather than those that are ego-based or imposed by society or their environment. This doesn't always mean that they will be happy, but by living with authenticity and grace and learning self-love, they should feel more at peace within themselves.

Taking a leap of faith – becoming the driver, not the passenger

There is no question that embracing a spiritual life usually requires some leaps of faith. It all comes down to whether your client continues to repeat patterns of be-haviour and experience psychological distress and fear, or whether they want to be freer from discomfort, pain, and suffering.

When clients take a leap of faith, this usually feels like they are jumping off the edge of a cliff without a parachute, not knowing whether they will land safely. It is learning to surrender to the fear that they have been holding on to that has been keeping them stuck repeating various life patterns or scenarios. Learning to make new choices and create a new template for their lives is ex-ceptionally challenging at times, especially at the beginning of therapy and again this is where encouragement and understanding of what your client is going through is imperative. Supporting clients in moving away from what is familiar to them, even if it is in horrendous experiences, can be frightening. Sometimes your client will feel a level of comfort in the familiar even if their experiences have been abusive or traumatic, feeling that it is 'better the devil you know!'

Usually these leaps of faith are there to show clients just that; when they take that leap they have to have faith that it will turn out alright without knowing what the outcome will be, what will happen and what support will be provided along the way. If they knew all of this information beforehand it wouldn't be a leap of faith! The only thing that prevents them from taking the leap will be their ego (or another's) convincing them that they are making a big mistake, highlighting all the things that could go wrong, and telling them how they need to cling to everything in their life to survive. Learning to live a life through the heart and/or soul provides the foundation on which to base their leaps of faith. While on their spiritual journey clients will probably have opportunities to take several leaps of faith, maybe in different areas of their life, for example, in work situations, relationships, and friendships. Helping your client learn to recognise when these opportunities are being presented to them is part way there to taking that leap; the more aware and resourced they are, the more confident they will feel in taking that jump.

My own experience of living life through my heart and soul

Being on a spiritual journey can be quite subtle or rather intense. For me, it was subtle to begin with and then I had a period of seven years that was extremely intense. I had many blocks and restrictions that stopped me from honouring my heart and soul, including issues of judgement, criticism, inadequacy, sense of duty and responsibility, trying to fit in with others rather than respect myself and so forth, and thus I would often try to please others to my own detriment. Reflecting back, I can identify certain moments when I was increasing my awareness of the impact that both people and environmental situations were having on me at a heart and soul level. One of those key times was when I had very young children and would attend baby groups and gatherings to entertain my children. I never really enjoyed these events because I found them rather superficial; I was aware on one level that the main commonality factor was the children. That isn't to say the parents were not lovely people, more that I just didn't have much in common with them and therefore didn't feel comfortable in myself, in other words I wasn't feeling like I was honouring my authentic self. When my eldest child was three years old I had arranged a joint birthday party with another family; I really didn't enjoy the experience at all, it made me feel drained and uncomfortable so I made a conscious decision that day that I did not have to keep trying to fit into the group anymore. While I knew that there would be some backlash to this, the relief I felt at having made this decision was immense. There have been many other occasions earlier in my life where I have been in situations where I did not feel comfortable; my body was telling me clearly when I was engaging in draining activities or with people who were not necessarily nurturing my heart and soul. In such situations, I sometimes thought 'I wonder whether if I got up and left would anyone would notice or care?' For many years I did not honour my heart and soul, I wasn't brave enough and I listened to my ego that created the fear, scared of being judged or criticised for doing what was authentic to me and what the consequences would be if I did not conform to others' expectations. I am now acutely aware of how my heart and soul communicate to me. I have also learned to be true to where my interests and passions lie, generally focusing on certain members of my family, close friends, work, spiritual journey, yoga, meditation, and quiet time. I am still shocked by the brutality and cruelty of how people can behave. However, I am learning to be more self-compassionate and grow in self-love so that I can be true to who I am and what feels right to me. I see these challenges now as opportunities to test out whether I can work toward authenticity and not get caught in ego battles, instead taking a step back, connecting with my heart and soul and responding from a place of compassion. The wonderful gift about facing my fears and working on letting go of my egoic thinking is that I no longer spend my time constantly striving to achieve what others want or expect from me. If I cannot be accepted and loved for the person I am, faults and all, then there is no place for such individuals in my life. This is a work in progress but the more I try to live an authentic life, the more content and peaceful I feel which enables me to live a life of ease and grace.

I have also been increasingly aware of my soul communicating with me when it was struggling or suffering. This has been more profound than listening to my heart, as my soul tends to really step in when a major decision needs to be made. There have been times when I could literally feel my soul dying; this has led me to make very big decisions (or new choices) to take those leaps of faith and to venture into unknown territory. For example, leaving a financially secure job to become self-employed and also making significant changes in my personal life. Hand on heart, while those choices were very challenging and frightening to make, when I listened to my soul and honoured what it was guiding me to do, I never had any regrets and never looked back. The freedom I felt and still feel is a confirmation to me that I made the right decisions.

Living life through your heart and soul – what to expect

During my life, I have had to face many deep fears. It has been a frightening and challenging journey and there have been times when I have questioned what I am doing and been close to giving up. I have also watched some close friends go through a similar process and while it is natural for them to seek support and reassurance and also for me to provide them assistance, I have had to be careful not to become the rescuer and prevent them from getting to that deepest place themselves so that they can rise to the beautiful light afterwards and discover their own authenticity.

The same is true for our clients. As therapists and clinicians we need to act from a place of compassionate support and understanding but not to act as rescuers. Rescuing others from their distress prevents them from learning that they are themselves strong enough to get through their own difficulties. This fine balance may be difficult to achieve, but using a spiritual perspective, the more aware you become of why and how you respond in certain situations with your clients, the more informed you are of whether to act or hold back. If in doubt, ask yourself the question:

> What is my client meant to learn from this experience or situation to help them to move forward?

We can also ask ourselves:
what am I meant to learn, teach or heal from supporting this client?
or,
what is this experience teaching me?
or,
what I am trying to teach or heal for my client?

I emphasise and also warn clients that embarking on a mindful spiritual journey may alter their perception of life around them. The more aware they become of themselves and what feels true from a heart and soul perspective, the harder it can feel to fit into an everyday 'normal' life. This isn't to deter anyone, but it is really important that clients are aware that their lives may change significantly, hopefully for the better, because they are becoming truer to themselves. It isn't unusual to find clients' friendships or interests change. Part of the process is letting go of all that no longer serves a purpose at a heart and soul level and instead learning to embrace that which nurtures them. This can happen quite subtly or very quickly depending on circumstances and spiritual openness. The more authentic a life that your client can live, hopefully the less suffering and distress they should experience.

Being open to the concept that as therapists and clinicians we can learn from every one of our clients is also opening ourselves up to grow stronger on our own individual life journeys. I learn so much from my clients; it is such an honour and a privilege every time someone is secure and safe enough to open up and be vulnerable with me and share their suffering and distress and I hope I will always hold this perspective and never take it for granted. I have learned gratitude, joy, appreciation, honour, courage, pride, compassion, integrity, and so much more from my clinical work. I can't imagine that I will ever stop learning and the more I learn, the more I have to give back in abundance.

Summary

- The aim of assisting clients to live an authentic life through their heart and soul is that it eases their psychological pain and suffering.
- Research findings have shown the benefits of working with clients at a heart-to-heart level where therapists spiritually resonate with their clients. Heartmath technology has shown positive physiological benefits of living life through the heart.
- Communications from the soul can present as opportunities to connect with the higher self and facilitate healing and may occur in different forms of 'knowing' or intuition, ranging from visual, auditory, kinaesthetic, proprioceptive, and direct knowing.
- Clients can start becoming aware of what enriches or drains them in life to make healthy changes as well as use positive referencing beliefs and affirmations.
- The Ful Trilogy is mindfulness, heartfulness and soulfulness. Learning to connect in all of these ways increases your client's awareness of what their heart and soul are trying to communicate to them and enables them to start taking the journey toward living an authentic life.
- Making new choices that are heart and soul led may require your client to take leaps of faith. This can be an exceptionally challenging but rewarding process.

Part 3

Heart Led Psychotherapy (HLP)

6

The stages of HLP

We carry inside of us the wonders we seek outside of us.

Rumi

Part 3 of this book focuses on the framework and process of HLP and how to imple-ment this with your clients. In this chapter, you will be guided through the stages of how to identify: the underlying challenges, traumas, and attachment/relationship difficulties, the resulting blocks and restrictions, and repeated themes and patterns that underlie your client's psychological distress. The role of the observer is then explained, which helps clients create a degree of detachment from a challenge in order to identify potential life lessons. The spiritually informed concept of life les-sons is detailed as it is central to HLP; that clients are on an individual journey and that challenges represent opportunities to experience and understand life lessons, enabling your client to enhance their ability to understand themselves and situa-tions more fully, develop self-love and authenticity. Ideas or themes of potential life lessons are provided as well as a discussion on the gifts that can be gained from living a heart and soul led life. Chapter 7 will show you how to explain HLP to cli-ents and includes suggested scripts that you can use, as well as case examples that illustrate the key areas of the model. The overall framework of HLP is the same for both the HL model and the HASL model and the main difference is that the HASL model includes the *additional* components of working at a soul level, which are discussed in more detail in Chapter 8.

Spiritual basis of HLP

The key concepts of HLP were discussed in Chapter 1. Some spiritual beliefs sug-gest that relationships formed, including family, friends, work colleagues, neigh-bours, acquaintances, or someone we meet for a brief time, present opportunities to *learn, teach and/or heal* (both ways). If a relationship is very challenging or de-structive, this may indicate blocks and restrictions from previous past life encoun-ters at a soul level (Weiss & Weiss, 2012). Sometimes, just using the HL model can empower clients to understand toxic or challenging relationships or situations

DOI: 10.4324/9781003613749-9

differently, by following the process of becoming the observer; understanding what the relationship or situation is trying to learn, teach, or heal in themselves or the other person and make new choices so that the dynamics change. If, in spite of this, these relationships or situations continue to be challenging and your client is open to spirituality and the presence of a soul, it may be beneficial to consider the HASL model. The HASL model includes the concept that blocks and restrictions may occur at a soul level and therefore offers the option of your client exploring additional soul level healing. Soul therapies are believed by some spiritual practitioners to help identify, clear and heal blocks and restrictions at a soul level, and this is discussed in more detail in Chapter 8. At the end of the day you have to work with your client's beliefs and what resonates with them.

HLP stages

Whether you are using the HL or HASL model, the structure to follow includes:

- Identifying current life challenges, traumas, and attachment/relationship difficulties.
- Identifying current life blocks and restrictions.
- Identifying current life repeated themes.
- Enabling clients to become aware of the impact of their ego.
- Helping clients to start becoming observers of the challenges they find themselves in.
- Identifying which potential life lessons clients are experiencing through their challenging situations.
- Helping clients to move their awareness into their heart and soul and start recognising what new choices they can make and what positives they can take away from challenges. This may require clients to take leaps of faith.

Figure 6.1 illustrates the HL model, which as I have already mentioned, is also the underlying framework for the HASL model (illustrated in Figure 8.1 in Chapter 8).

Identifying challenges, traumas, and attachment/ relationship difficulties

The first stage in HLP is to identify specific challenges, traumas and attachment/ relationship difficulties that have occurred during a client's history. I always start my initial assessment by being curious about what has brought the person to come and seek therapy at this stage in their life:

- What are the current issues that they are struggling with?
- How are these current issues impacting on their daily life?
- What current challenges are they facing that make life difficult?

Challenges, trauma and attachment difficulties

Blocks and restrictions

Repeated patterns of behaviour or situations   EGO   EGO

EGO   Psychological distress

Becoming the observer

Identify what life lessons can be experienced

EGO   HEART

Make same choices   Make new choices

Attain gifts

Self-love and authenticity

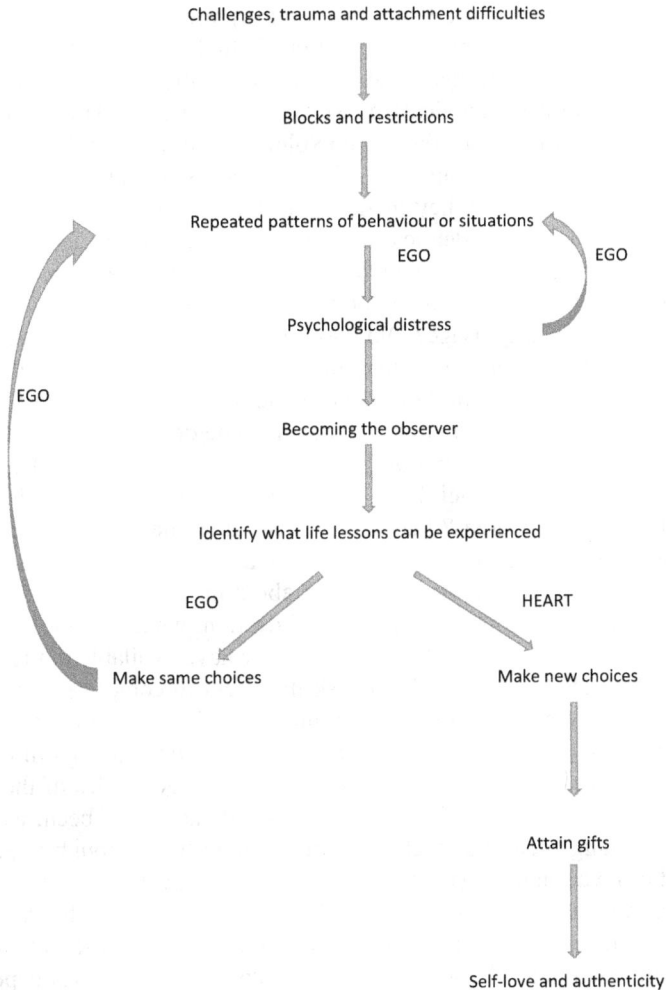

Figure 6.1 The Heart Led model

- Are these challenges specific to selected areas of their life or affecting every aspect of their life?
- What are their current relationships like with other people, for example, family, friends, work colleagues, neighbours, or peer group?

Once I have gathered this information I complete a detailed background history. I want to find out about the client's early attachment history and relationships formed with their parents/carers and other key family members or significant people in their life, including teachers or people in their community. Completing a genogram with clients (which includes all significant family members – parents, grandparents, aunts and uncles, siblings, and children) is highly informative as it enables you to explore valuable information about family members who may also have difficulties (medical or psychological), as well as the nature of relationships between different members. I then do a thorough exploration of the client's developmental and educational history, keeping note of any absences or lapses in their memory. I am keen to know whether they made friendships, whether there is a history of bullying or trauma, what academic qualifications they achieved, and what age they left formal education. I explore when their difficulties such as anxiety or depression first started and how these impacted on their life: is there a history of self-harm, alcohol, smoking, or drug usage? Did they receive any therapeutic support or did their difficulties go un-noticed? If they did receive support, what kind of support was offered and was this helpful or not? Depending on the age of the client, I then discuss what working opportunities they had in some detail.

Throughout all of this exploration I am making note of how the client reacts to discussing various areas of their life – do they become tearful or withdrawn, or resistant to discussing any areas? I am also curious about details of positive times in their life, as these are important areas that can be used later when resource building. Toward the end of the assessment, I inquire about their sleep and eating patterns, any medication they are taking, any suicidal ideation, what activities and hobbies they are participating in, what social support they have available to them and also what are their goals for therapy. I may ask the client to complete some questionnaires, such as assessing for dissociation, mood, anxiety, and trauma. If there are any opportunities to explore their spiritual ideas and beliefs then I will incorporate these within my assessment. Overall, I want to have a good idea of the person in the room with me; what have their experiences and challenges been, what is their reason for wanting their life to change and do they have enough psychological insight and motivation to engage therapeutically? Amongst all of this exploration, perhaps the most important factor is whether the client can develop a therapeutic relationship and I work extremely hard at building up their trust so that they can feel safe and contained. The assessment may take several sessions depending on the client's experiences, attachment history and trauma, but nothing will be possible if a therapeutic relationship cannot be built. I have discussed the concept of taking an 'energetic' approach to one's clinical work, therapeutic relationship and one's personal life in a lot more detail elsewhere (Dent, 2025).

Identifying the blocks and restrictions

The main source of blocks and restrictions often occurs as a result of significant relationships in your client's life. Any complex relationships are indicators of blocks and restrictions that may have occurred in this lifetime. If a client has experienced attachment difficulties growing up, possible blocks and restrictions would include negative beliefs such as not believing they deserve happiness, are unlovable, or not good enough. They may therefore have difficulty in trusting others and do not feel they can show their emotions. They are likely to have shut down and dissociated from their emotions, or have put up a brick wall to protect themselves because they would not have felt contained or secure.

Traumatic or significant life events can also result in blocks and restrictions, for example, if your client was in an accident, experienced or witnessed abuse, or was bullied at school or at work. Any environment that your client has encountered, whether it is home, school, work, community, or extracurricular events or holidays, can represent places where difficulties occurred. If this has happened, clients may avoid situations or people that remind them of such events, or become hypervigilant in certain situations or around certain people. Any unprocessed trauma can easily be triggered by sounds, sight, smells, touch, and taste without your client being aware of this. Noticing how your client responds in sessions when discussing their background history can also provide indications of unprocessed traumas, for example, if they become tearful or distressed or anxious when relaying some information to you. Sometimes information arises beyond the initial assessment, so it is important to adopt an open and aware approach and be ready and able to incorporate this into what has already been gathered in your formulation.

Identifying repeated patterns of behaviour and recurrent themes

Once the blocks and restrictions have been identified, the next stage is to determine what impact these have had throughout your client's life. This is where it is important to consider the following questions:

- What are the current themes that your client is struggling with that are making life difficult?
- Are there any similarities between the current themes and previous challenges, traumas and attachment/relationship difficulties?
- Are these themes specific to certain areas of your client's life, or affecting every aspect of their life?

Repeated themes are often indicators of blocks and restrictions that have occurred for example:

- Are they constantly self-sacrificing and not getting their needs met?
- Do their underlying negative beliefs impact on the choices they are making in their life?
- Do they struggle to believe they can have happiness, peace, faith or trust in others or themselves?
- Do they constantly find themselves in very destructive relationships rather than harmonious partnerships?
- Have they not received love or positivity through their early life experiences and relationships and has this affected subsequent relationships?

- Do they feel trapped in relationships that are draining but cannot find a way to make changes?
- Is money a repeated issue – either believing they are not worthy, or struggling to hold on to something when it is going well?
- Do they self-sabotage?

If an individual has had very difficult early attachment relationships, one of the repeated themes they may experience is struggling to have intimate or emotionally close relationships with others, instead remaining detached and finding it hard to experience positive emotions because these feel unfamiliar and frightening to them. This will then impact on future attachments they form and they may remain numb, anxious, or depressed as a consequence (as well as other difficulties). Sometimes such individuals may find future partners or friends who are able to show them love and nurturance. These illustrate the significance of the other individuals acting as teachers or healers. The key area here is whether the client is able to internalise and experience this positive relationship. For example, I see many adult clients who have had very poor attachment relationships growing up and have learned to shut down their emotional responses as a survival strategy, which creates blocks and restrictions. The clients then meet someone who is able to offer them love and provide a nurturing and supportive relationship. This other individual is trying to teach the client that they can experience fulfilling relationships as well as try to heal past traumas and blocks and restrictions. While this is a positive aspect of their life, more often than not clients still find it immensely difficult to open up and receive love and affection from others. They may continue to believe that they are worthless, undeserving, not good enough and unlovable. Despite positively managing to maintain a relationship with someone, their ability to accept the positive emotions from their partner or children can still be impaired. On this level they are still stuck in the repeated themes or repeated patterns of behaviour.

Another indicator of clients having repeated themes is when they present in a resistant or emotionally detached manner in the therapeutic relationship. Their protective wall is there to keep them safe, so trying to engage in a session will probably make them feel uncomfortable and frightened. Just being in a session with you could make your client feel out of their emotional window of tolerance range, especially if you are engaging them with compassion and kindness. I have had a few clients tell me that they find my nurturing and compassionate approach uncomfortable or unfamiliar. If this happens, I thank them for their honesty and then give them an understanding as to why they feel this, so that they can learn to understand rather than see this as a problem. I explain that part of my work is to help them to feel more comfortable so that, with time, they can learn to experience the positive effect of our therapeutic relationship. I will then gently and consciously titrate how I am energetically in sessions to allow time for them to build up enough internal resources to be able to internalise positive affect.

During the process of identifying repeated themes, it is also important to try and find any positive situations where your client has made new choices that have resulted in a change of direction from the earlier repeated themes. Some positive areas to look out for include:

- What facilitated the new choice – was it a new partner, another significant individual or situation, or a change in social setting or circumstance?
- Were the new choices made from their heart and soul, which is more in line with their authentic selves?
- To what extent did making a new choice result in a different outcome?
- Are there any blocks and restrictions that are preventing your client from maximising what they can achieve from making new choices?

With practise, noticing repeated themes and patterns of behaviour gets easier and easier. The greater the depth of spiritual understanding of the therapist, the stronger their intuition and the more rapidly they can become aware of such repeated themes and patterns of their clients.

Becoming the observer, not the observed

This is a fundamental part of the model. It encourages clients to metaphorically step outside of the situation or challenge that they are finding themselves in, view the situation as an observer and then reflect on what is actually happening in an objective way, without being caught up in the dynamics. Only at this point can your client start to try to understand how this challenge is an opportunity to understand a particular life lesson. It is like asking your client to press the pause button on a film or a scene in a play, become the observer and start noticing what is happening with a degree of detachment. More often than not, when clients find themselves in challenges, they adopt the role of the victim and feel hard done by and possibly feel someone else or the situation is trying to punish them. They become so caught up in the drama or scene that they cannot reflect clearly, as their distress is too overwhelming. Metaphorically stepping outside and being the observer allows the client to feel more removed from the situation and thus enables them to reflect with clarity and composure.

How to help your clients become the observer

1   Teaching mindfulness

Mindfulness was discussed in detail in Chapter 4. Mindfulness is awareness, so the more mindful your client can become, the more aware they will be of recognising when they find themselves in challenges. This will then help them to follow the process of 'stepping outside' of the challenge and observe, reflect, learn, and take action. The quicker your client becomes aware of when they are caught in challenges, the quicker they become the observer, learn lessons, make new choices and experience less distress and suffering.

2   Help your client to recognise when they are identifying as the victim

Difficult encounters with others or situations are typically very painful and challenging. This can make a person feel that they are the victim of others' behaviour or wrong-doing and indeed sometimes they really have been the victim. The difficulty comes when the client's ego maintains the victim role long after the trauma, because it maintains the psychological distress. This is not a judgement or a criticism, merely a reflection of what typically happens. I myself have adopted this position many times in my life, sometimes I could argue justifiably, sometimes perhaps not. Regardless of the circumstances, when your client identifies with the victim role, they feel a sense of powerlessness to change themselves or the situation and are not able to see clearly what they can learn from this experience. They become stuck and feel helpless. Learning to become the victor gives your client a sense of strength and power to look at what needs changing for their benefit and that of others so that they can make new choices and stop repeating themes.

3   Letting go of the ego

Several exercises to help clients to let go of their ego were provided in Chapter 3. Mindfulness will also make them much more aware of when their ego is present and having an impact on their distress. As you ask your client to take the observer role, be aware of how they respond, and whether observations are coming from their ego, heart, or soul. If they are coming from their ego, sensitively help them to notice this; the ego will be clever and convincing and will put up a fight. Be patient and compassionate with your client as it may take them a while to learn to differentiate between their egoic thinking and their heart or soul messages.

4   Honouring the heart and soul

Encourage your client to learn to honour what their heart or soul is trying to communicate to them rather than their ego. You could use some of the exercises mentioned in Chapter 3 or Chapter 5. When your client honours what their heart or soul is communicating to them, they will be able to identify what they are to learn or experience from the challenges. This greater understanding will give them the ability to identify what new choices they can make.

Identifying the life lessons

It has already been discussed in Chapter 1 that some spiritual views and beliefs propose the concept of life lessons. HLP utilises this concept, understanding life as being an individual journey in which there are opportunities to experience different life lessons to provide a pathway to assist your client to express themselves with authenticity and self-love. Life lessons tend to be extremely difficult. As clients fully experience and understand their life lesson/s and work successfully on challenges and make the right choices, they may find that they are less likely to experience challenges with the same theme. If they get stuck, or continue to make egoic choices, they may find that certain challenges increase in order to help them with their understanding of their life lesson and make different choices that are heart and soul led. The critical point to remember is that as your client gains a level of knowledge and understanding about what they are meant to be experiencing, this may ultimately enable them to make new choices and live a more authentic life.

Life lessons can affect your client in specific life areas or all aspects of their life. For example, they may affect work, finances, significant relationships, health, personal growth, spirituality, friendships, family, hobbies and interests, environment, or systems. Life lessons are not there because your client is being punished. Nor are they something that your client must achieve in order to 'learn' or 'grow' because they are lacking in some way. It is believed that the experience that clients can gain through the life lesson may enhance their ability to understand situations and themselves more fully and will guide them to make more informed choices that are heart and soul led rather than ego-led. In order to conceptualise life lessons and how they impact on your client, I have broken them down into four headings; primary, joint, everyday, and systemic life lessons. Again, this is based on certain spiritual beliefs rather than conclusive facts.

Primary life lessons

Your clients will have a primary life lesson and possibly one or a few secondary life lessons and they will encounter situations or challenges in order to help them experience these lessons, so that they can be more authentic in how they choose to live their life. Life lessons tend to be extremely difficult and clients may have spent many, many lifetimes working on these lessons, or they may just choose to experience a theme for a particular lifetime. As clients fully experience and understand their life lesson/s and work successfully on challenges and make the right choices, they are less likely to find themselves in challenges with the same theme. Once a life lesson has been completed, the client no longer needs to have those experiences related to that life lesson; they have experienced this fully. If they get stuck, or if they have done a lot of healing work but do not take advantage of opportunities or continue to make egoic choices, they may find that challenges will increase in order to help them with their understanding of their life lesson. This in turn will encourage them to make the right choices that are heart and soul led. It is not always essential to complete a life lesson; sometimes a soul will decide that they have gained enough understanding and that they do not need to continue with a particular lesson, but decide to move on to something else, or focus on their joint lessons and everyday life challenges. The critical point to remember is that as your client gains a level of knowledge and understanding about what they are meant to be experiencing, this will ultimately enable them to make new choices and live a more authentic life.

Joint lessons

Most clients will have a few additional joint lessons with other people, especially if the other person is very significant in their life, for example, a family member or close friend. These joint lessons provide an opportunity to work on a slightly different theme to their primary life lesson in order to learn, teach, or heal with another person. Joint lessons can be present just for this lifetime, or can be carried over from previous lifetimes if it is felt that the learning process is incomplete and further work in that area would be beneficial.

Joint lessons and being the 'Rescuer'

It is not uncommon for clients to try and rescue others from their challenges and the associated learning, as they do not like seeing others struggle or suffer. While their intentions may be honourable, the difficulty with this is that this is comes from their ego, believing the other person needs their help, but in fact they are stopping the other person from learning and progressing for themselves. Sometimes this is also done as a deflection and avoidance of having to face working on their own life lesson. The important thing to keep reminding your client is that it is an INDI-VIDUAL journey so they need to keep focused on their lessons rather than trying to rescue others on their journey.

Everyday life lessons

In addition to your client's primary/secondary and joint lessons, they are likely to encounter everyday opportunities to experience different lessons. Interactions with other people, no matter how short in duration, are always opportunities to learn, teach or heal. Clients may notice a period of time in which there is a common theme to the issues or challenges they are experiencing, this will be occurring to broaden their understanding beyond their main life lessons.

Systemic life lessons

I have already discussed how life lessons can potentially affect us at an individual level. However, they may also impact on us at a systemic level too. I would there-fore like to highlight how major traumas can present as opportunities for life les-sons to be experienced on a larger systemic basis and have provided two such cases below to illustrate this point.

Stephen Lawrence's death in 1993

Stephen Lawrence was brutally and horrifically murdered in 1993 because of the colour of his skin and his death shook the nation. Trying to understand how anything positive can come from such an awful act seems unimaginable.

I was listening to the radio in April 2018 and on the news, they announced that after 25 years Stephen's father, Neville Lawrence, had come to a place of forgiveness for the murderers who took his precious and beloved first son from this life. He said that it was the hardest thing he had ever had to do. He reached this place despite there being no remorse from his son's murderers, because his Christian faith had given him the strength to do this. As I listened to this announcement, I wondered from an HLP perspective whether forgiveness may be his life lesson and I felt immense pride that he could find such compassion for the murderers of his son, having gone through such an awful experience. Systemically the death of Stephen Lawrence had an impact at a national level, resulting in social change, with an increase in awareness of racial issues, which led to organisations being created to help people understand and act against racism.

Manchester bombings in 2017

If we consider traumas involving more individuals such as the Manchester bombing in the UK in 2017, it is again hard to think about what positives can be derived from these atrocious events. While there will be an impact on each of the individuals involved, there was also a larger impact on the community and nation. Very quickly, the local community in and around Manchester worked together to manage the impact of this trauma – local people were opening up their doors with offers of help and support, including accommodation and food, local taxi drivers made sure people got home safely, acts of kindness were multiple. On a larger scale, a memorial concert was quickly organised to raise money to support those immediately affected by the event. The bombers may have felt that the bomb would have caused division and destruction in the UK, but the message that arose from this trauma was paramount and clear 'Together we stand as one.' Rather than have the intended effect, it brought people closer and stronger as a unit.

Here are some of the potential themes for life lessons. This list is not exhaustive and I am finding that I am adding to it all the time as I work with clients in this way:

- Abundance, acceptance, accountability, achievement, acknowledgement, appreciation, approval, assertiveness.
- Balance, beauty, blessing, bliss, boldness.
- Caring, centredness, charity, commitment, compassion, confidence, consciousness, consideration, contentment, cooperation, courage.
- Decisiveness, dependability, deserving, determination, discernment, Divine Love.

- Ease, empowerment, energy, enthusiasm.
- Faith, flexibility, forgiveness, fulfilment.
- Generosity, giving, grace, gratitude, growth.
- Happiness, harmony, healing, honesty, humility.
- Independence, inner-authority, inspiration, integrity, intuition.
- Joy.
- Kindness, knowledge.
- Laughter, learning, light-heartedness, listening, love, loyalty.
- Mercy, mindfulness, moderation.
- Openness.
- Partnership, passion, patience, peace, perseverance, persistence, pleasure, possibility, power, practice, presence, protection.
- Receiving, recognition, reflection, reward.
- Safety, satisfaction, security, self-acceptance, self-assurance, self-belief, self-care, self-determination, self-love, self-worth, sensitivity, sincerity, spirituality, strength, success, surrender.
- Temperance, tenacity, trust, truth.
- Unconditionality, understanding.
- Vulnerability.
- Well-being, wisdom.

Themes can be experienced in both positive and negative forms, take for example the theme of power. This could be related to when to exhibit power and when not to be so powerful, or when to allow others to be powerful or not. Each theme therefore can have several messages to portray, and in different areas of a client's life and with different types of relationships, but all of these are important to allow the soul to fully express its true nature.

Receiving is one of the everyday themes that I personally have had to work on throughout my life, which has involved learning to be open to receiving kindness, support, and love from others. Sometimes I may have been given a present, either at a particular occasion (Christmas or birthdays) or for no particular reason other than someone wanting to show kindness to me. This has been quite a challenge for me to accept and receive because I had an underlying belief that I didn't deserve such kindness and love. However, I am learning with time to say thank you and receive unconditionally. It has been hard to do this without believing or feeling that I need to repay someone back for their generosity. With time I have also learned to be open to receiving offers of support, either through friendship or practical support, as well as learning to ask for help instead of believing I have to do everything myself. By learning to feel more comfortable with receiving, I am also allowing the other individual to enjoy the experience of giving. I have also had to learn when not to receive, especially if something is being said or given to me in an unauthentic or egocentric way.

When I am working with clients, I become curious as to what a client's life lesson/s could be. Table 6.1 provides some potential ideas that link recurrent themes or presenting issues with various life lessons. This table is just to be

Table 6.1 Potential ideas that link psychological issues with various life lessons

Presenting issue or recurrent theme	Life lesson
Depression, isolation, lack of joy	Empowerment, self-determination, courage, compassion, kindness, forgiveness, faith, trust, happiness, joy, strength, beauty, gratitude, bliss, laughter, blessing, appreciation, joy
Criticism, abuse	Truth, self-determination, assertiveness, self-worth, understanding, strength, safety, self-love
Being in unhappy or unrewarding situations	Self-belief, self-worth, autonomy, empowerment, achievement, recognition, inner-authority, approval, assertiveness, success
Trauma, loss	Forgiveness, compassion, courage, strength, self-belief, healing, Divine love
Acting for one's own needs and desires without recognising the impact on others	Integrity, courage, honour, honesty, truth, generosity, kindness, compassion, spirituality, humility, cooperation
Blaming others, victimisation	Mercy, Divine love, consciousness, accountability, understanding, humility, awareness, grace, empathy, acknowledgement, charity, wisdom
Destructive or unfulfilling relationships	Peace, harmony, partnership, forgiveness, compassion, strength, empowerment, self-worth, self-belief, possibility
Anxiety, worry, fear, doubt	Faith, trust, patience, ease, contentment, security, spirituality, safety, confidence, empowerment, strength, determination, surrender, acceptance
Misunderstanding, judgement, failure, self-sabotage,	Compassion, clarity, self-belief, mercy, self-worth, deserving, understanding, giving, persistence, sensitivity
Obedience, timidity	Self-determination, self-worth, empowerment, courage, independence, cooperation, persistence, inspiration, receiving
Guilt, shame	Forgiveness, self-belief, self-worth, blessing, happiness, deserving, gratitude, compassion, pleasure, fulfilment, healing
Addictions	Moderation, tolerance, honesty, deserving, faith, sincerity, abundance

used as an example and is not definitive. Be curious and explore different possibilities as you see fit, based on your client's experiences and the difficulties they have had with making new choices. Remember, your client may be working on a number of different life lessons including primary life lessons and possibly some secondary life lessons, joint lessons and everyday life lessons due to ongoing challenges.

Identifying the gift

Each and every challenge, whether it is big or small can provide a gift. This will usually be by truly experiencing and understanding a life lesson to enable the client to be more aligned to their authentic self and experience self-love. This idea can be particularly difficult for some people to conceptualise initially, because they are so caught up with being the victim that they are failing to recognise that something good can come out of every situation. When life lessons are experienced and understood, new choices can be made to break out of the repeated themes that have previously been occurring and the pathway on the individual life journey becomes smoother. When new choices are made that are in keeping with what your clients' heart and souls desire, rather than their ego, the gift within this is to experience more fulfilment, forgiveness, freedom and gratitude and live life with ease and grace rather than distress and turmoil.

During particularly difficult challenges, it is likely that your client may need to take a leap of faith in a situation in order to achieve the gift. This occurs when clients understand a particular life lesson and are ready to make a new heart and soul led choice. Taking the leap of faith has previously been discussed in Chapter 5 but can be exceptionally challenging in itself – your client may experience extreme fear because the outcome is uncertain. However, once leaps of faith have been taken, your client will hopefully begin to feel gratitude for their experiences regardless of how painful they have been. They may feel inspired and have the courage and strength to make changes in their life that feel genuine and true to them when faced with future challenges. Your client may notice a sense of freedom, as they are no longer constrained by repeated themes and blocks and restrictions and they begin to learn to have self-love, self-compassion, self-belief, self-acceptance, and self-worth.

Everyday life lessons and gifts

In my sessions with clients, I am increasingly noticing many opportunities to apply HLP to their everyday life challenges. If clients already have a good understanding of HLP and if I am flexible with the structure of my sessions, we can explore everyday life challenges that have arisen between sessions if required. The benefits of this include helping them to gain an increased awareness, empowerment and understanding about their challenges, as well as feeling more resourced to tackle further situations as they arise. Usually these conversations happen when events between sessions have occurred that make the client feel completely overwhelmed and exhausted. By reflecting on these challenges and applying HLP, clients often come back at the next session reporting a sense of relief and freedom when they have managed to make new choices; this is part of the gifts they receive as a consequence of their actions.

Summary

- The framework of HLP underpins both the HL model and the HASL model.
- It is important to complete a detailed history with your client in order to identify their challenges, traumas and attachment/relationship difficulties.
- The next stage is to identify what your client's blocks and restrictions are as well as repeated themes throughout their life.
- Strategies to help clients become observers include learning mindfulness, recognising when they are in the victim role, learning to let go of their ego and start honouring their heart and soul.
- The spiritual concept of life lessons is central to HLP. Challenges are seen as opportunities to experience life lessons that will enable your client to enhance their ability to understand themselves and situations more fully.
- Life lessons are believed to provide opportunities to learn, teach or heal.
- A client may be working on a primary life lesson, possibly a few secondary life lessons and some joint lessons with other individuals with whom they have a significant relationship.
- In addition, your client may encounter everyday or systemic life lessons from time to time, which will provide further opportunities to experience different themes.
- Clients can work toward receiving the gifts from challenging situations, by starting to enjoy a more fulfilled, freer life with a sense of gratitude, forgiveness, inspiration, self-love, self-worth, self-acceptance, self-compassion, and self-belief.

7

Teaching clients HLP

Your heart knows the way. Run in that direction.

Rumi

The previous chapter discussed the different stages of HLP. This chapter will focus on the process of how to teach your clients HLP, including a flowchart that you can follow. Suggested scripts are provided for you to use to explain the process to clients along with case examples to illustrate the different stages of HLP. Two exercises are also provided: the first helps your client to learn how to apply HLP to re-write earlier challenges in their life so that they gain a better understanding of how these have been opportunities to experience life lessons. The second exercise is teaching the client how to re-write current life challenges using HLP.

Teaching clients the process of HLP

Figure 7.1 provides a flowchart of HLP for you to follow. Once you have done a thorough assessment, you should be ready to share your formulation with your client as to what is likely to be causing their psychological distress based on their challenges and traumas, blocks and restrictions and repeated themes. Having determined your client's spiritual beliefs this informs you of which HLP model to use. I use the script below before showing them a diagram of either the HL model (Figure 6.1 in Chapter 6) or HASL model (Figure 8.1 in Chapter 8) to talk them through the process, incorporating my formulation to determine whether this resonates with them. Please adapt the script depending on which model you are using, referring just to 'heart' or 'heart and soul' if using the HL model and referring to 'heart and soul' if you are using the HASL model where your client is open to the idea of reincarnation.

Here is a simple way of teaching HLP to clients:

Life can be considered an individual journey in which we have opportunities to understand and experience life lessons. Life lessons are opportunities to learn, teach or heal others and ourselves. We all have our own individual primary life lesson and sometimes a few secondary life lessons, which are the key lessons

DOI: 10.4324/9781003613749-10

Complete detailed assessment. Provide an HLP formulation to your client (based on challenges, traumas and significant relationships, blocks and restrictions, repeated themes that lead to psychological distress).

Is your client spiritual?

NO   **YES**

Use Heart Led (HL) model.

Use Heart and Soul Led (HASL) model.

Explain about life lessons. Introduce HLP and the HL model diagram.

Explain about life lessons. Introduce HLP and the HASL model diagram. Discuss the idea of soul level blocks and restrictions and the option of soul therapies.

Teach client about the ego and ways to let go of the ego.

Teach client the process of becoming the observer.

HL model   **HASL model**

Explore potential life lessons where clients connect with their heart.

Explore potential life lessons where clients connect with their heart and soul.

Teach clients the value of making new HL choices and leaps of faith, identify the gifts and live a more authentic life.

Teach clients the value of making new HASL choices and leaps of faith, identify the gifts and live a more authentic life.

Encourage clients to use HLP with all challenges in their life.

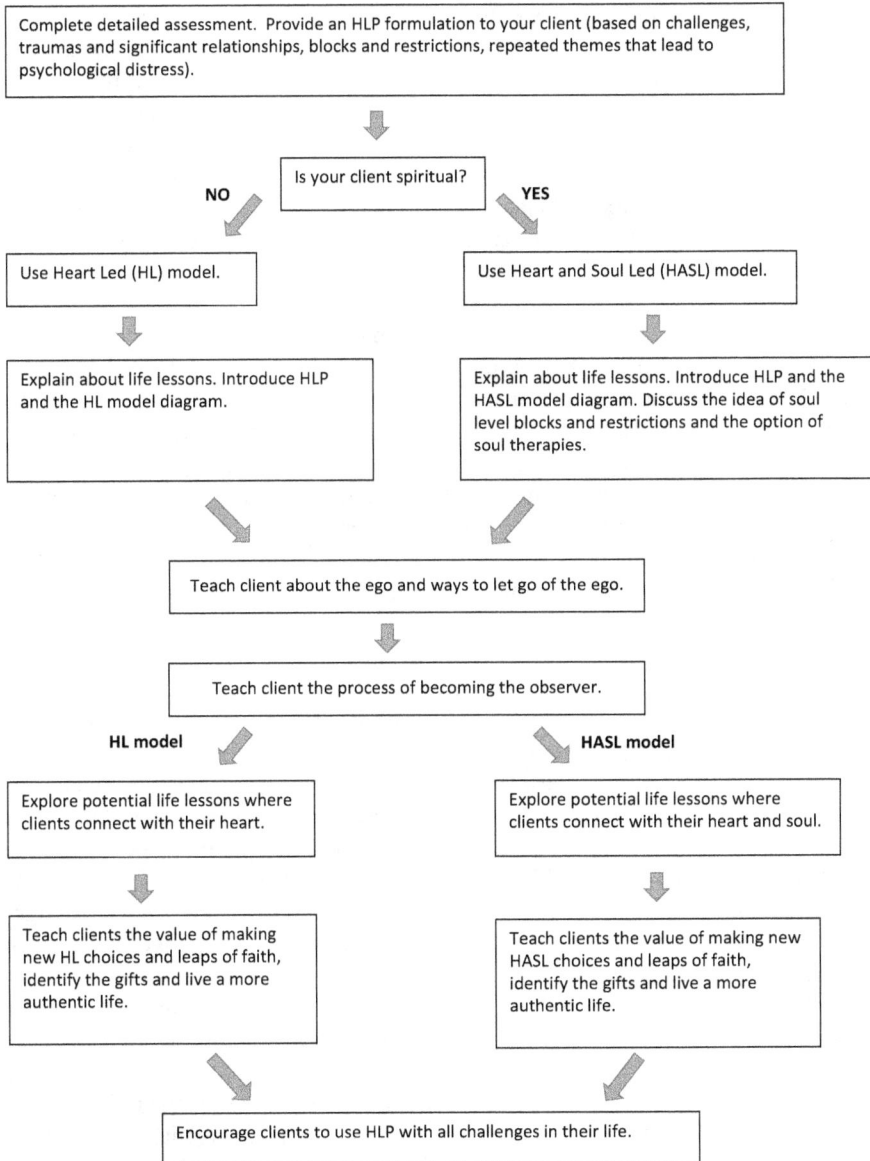

Figure 7.1 Flowchart of Heart Led Psychotherapy

we are trying to really understand throughout our lives. Examples of life lessons include abundance, empowerment, forgiveness, compassion, and so forth. Life lessons are meant to be experienced in many different ways and in both positive and negative forms. Take for example the theme of courage. This could be learning when to have courage and when not to have courage, or when to allow others to be courageous or not. Life lessons may affect just a few aspects of our life, or all areas, including work, primary relationships, family, friends, hobbies, health and well-being, spirituality, and our place in the community or our environment. In addition to our primary life lesson, we also may have joint lessons with a few significant people in our lives in which we are working jointly with them to try and teach, heal or learn a particular theme. In addition, we have everyday life lessons that are opportunities to experience a wider range of attributes or themes to help us broaden and develop as individuals and to ultimately gain the most out of life. For example, you may go through a phase in life where lots of challenges are happening in different areas of your life but have a similar theme, for example, assertiveness. Finally, there are systemic life lessons that can be experienced where an event or trauma impacts at either a community, national or global level and this provides another opportunity to work on additional themes beyond the primary, joint or everyday life lessons. It is important to keep remembering that we are on an individual journey. It can be really tempting at times to try and help others, but we have to remember that if we try and 'rescue' them, even if our intentions are honourable, we are stopping them from learning their own lessons and this also takes our attention away from our own journey.

We may all have had challenges in our life when we encounter difficult relationships with family members, friends or other people. This can make us believe that we are unlovable, that we don't deserve happiness, or that we are to blame or not good enough. We may also have found ourselves in difficult situations or traumatic experiences, possibly at school, in our neighbourhood or at work, which could make us feel a failure, inadequate or powerless. All of these challenges can greatly affect us and when such difficulties occur and are not resolved, they become blocks and restrictions. Carrying these blocks and restrictions around with us makes it really hard when we have new challenges to face and we then often find ourselves repeating similar challenges and experiences throughout our lives.

Although it can be very hard to recognise at the time, something positive can come from every difficult challenge that will enable us to understand the situation more clearly. A technique that can be used to break out of this repeated cycle is to learn to look at challenges in a different way and see them as opportunities to understand or experience something. This can change how we manage the challenge and can help lead to a different and more positive outcome. For example, if you have been in a difficult relationship it may be an opportunity for you to learn to be empowered, or to have courage or strength, so that you don't allow someone to treat you again in a hurtful or abusive way. I would like to show you a model from a therapy called Heart Led Psychotherapy that provides a way of understanding challenges as opportunities to experience life lessons.

At this point I introduce either the diagram of the HL or HASL model and talk the client through the stages *up until* the psychological distress, personalising to their situation so that it makes it real to them. I then introduce the topic of the ego (previously described in Chapter 3), as this is fundamental to the model. I am repeating the script again so that you can see how it fits in with the HLP process.

> The ego keeps us stuck in a repetitive cycle of repeated patterns of behaviour and maintains psychological distress. There is a general acceptance that we all have an ego. When I talk about the ego I am not referring to being narcissistic or self-righteous. Instead I am referring to that part of us that creates our thoughts and desires and expectations. Our ego is very clever, it hooks us into people or situations because it makes us believe that we need these things in order to function or survive, but this creates dependency and we stop believing that we can function without such things. Our ego makes us both judge and feel judged or criticised, makes us take the blame for difficulties, or feel responsible for everyone else's happiness except our own. The problem is that when we live life through our ego we often end up repeating patterns of behaviour or situations and this makes us feel stuck and trapped. We are never happy with what we do have because we are always searching for something else. Our ego doesn't want to be ignored so it provides very good arguments as to why we should stay stuck in challenging or difficult circumstances. Our ego creates FEAR about change, convincing us that something bad will happen if we make new choices – this is its biggest weapon.

This is the stage where I explain about learning to become the observer.

> Life lessons are usually really difficult to experience and often we feel consumed by them and get caught up in the challenge. It is so easy to start feeling like a victim of the experience, which makes us feel powerless and vulnerable, but it is our ego that is making us feel this way. Learning to step outside of the challenge and become the observer of challenges provides an opportunity to reflect on what is happening and helps us to view the situation differently; with some detachment and more clarity. It helps us to start understanding what the challenges are trying to teach us, identify what the life lesson is, so that we can make new choices instead of repeating similar themes or patterns in our lives that are ego based. We become the victor rather than the victim, which gives us strength and determination to tackle situations or people differently.
>
> At this important stage we have a choice to make. We could make the same choices which are from our ego, but the difficulty with making ego choices is that they keep us stuck in the repeated patterns of behaviour and this maintains our distress and suffering. On the other hand, we can learn how to make new choices that feel right at a heart (and soul) level. Heart (and soul) led choices can be very hard to make and sometimes this requires us to take a leap of faith. This can feel frightening, as if we are jumping off a cliff with no parachute and not knowing whether we would land safely or not. However, if we knew the outcome it wouldn't be a leap of faith! When choices are made that honour our heart (and soul) rather than our ego, they are more likely to lead

to positive outcomes and we can start to attain gifts; by this I mean a sense of gratitude, inspiration, freedom or truth and learn how to have self-love, self-belief, self-compassion, self-worth, and self-acceptance. We then start living a more authentic life.

Ask your client to give you some feedback as to whether this model resonates with them and their experiences. It may also be helpful to spend more time teaching your client about the power of the ego, how to utilise mindfulness in their life and how to learn to move their awareness into their heart. This has previously been explained in Chapters 3, 4, and 5 with exercises that you can tailor to your client's needs.

Teaching clients to become the observer

When you teach your client how to become an observer it is helpful to ask them to bring to mind a challenge they have experienced, either in their past or something that is current. I would then use the following script to show them how to become an observer of the challenge:

> I would like you to bring to mind that challenge that has been distressing for you. Imagine it is like being part of a play or drama where you are one of the ac-tors in the play or drama. Once you have clearly connected with that challenge, imagine pressing the pause button to just stop or freeze what is happening. Now I would like you to metaphorically imagine yourself stepping out of the play or drama and become the observer.

Once your client has become the observer, ask them the following relevant questions:

- What do you observe happening in this situation?
- What do you notice happening between individuals in this situation?
- What do you understand is the significance of certain individuals within this challenge?
- Do you see yourself as a victim in this challenge and feel punished or hard done by?
- What is your ego telling you about the situation or challenge that you are observing?
- What is your heart (and soul) trying to communicate to you about the situation or challenge that you are observing?
- How does it make you feel taking the role of the observer?

Spend some time exploring their answers to the questions you have posed to them, again taking care to identify whether any observations appear to be ego based, and if so, gently bring this to their awareness and see whether they can try to observe from their heart (and soul). This can take practise (for both you and your client) but remember the traits of the ego! If responses appear to be based on fear, expectations, hooks or the victim role, or any judgements or criticism then it is highly likely to be an ego answer.

Teaching clients to identify the life lessons

Having helped your client to become the observer to a particular challenge, now is the opportunity to reflect and wonder together what their life lesson/s could be. You as a therapist are not meant to know the exact answer for them; usually your client will be able to give some ideas of what they think their lessons may be. This is how I introduce this stage:

> Now that you are the observer of this challenge or situation, what I would like you to consider, at a heart (and soul) level, is what this situation is trying to help you to understand or experience. What do you think the life lesson may be about?

Some clients come up with ideas quite quickly. If they are struggling, use your intuition based on what you know about the client and their repeated themes and suggest potential ideas to see whether any resonate with them at a heart (and soul) level. You could look at some of the ideas presented in Table 6.1 to act as a guide, while recognising that this table is not exhaustive and can be expanded upon as required. Sometimes a theme of a life lesson becomes more apparent over the course of a few sessions. Be mindful to work from the heart (and soul) and not the ego!

Exploring the gifts gained and how to live more authentically

This final stage of HLP is exploring the following questions with your clients:

- How can you use the gained knowledge and understanding of your life lesson to take away something positive from the challenges you have experienced?
- How can you apply this gained knowledge and wisdom moving forward when you encounter new challenges?
- Are there any leaps of faith you may need to take to make heart and soul led choices and if so what would these be?
- What coping strategies and resources do you need to support you in taking any leaps of faith?
- Does making heart and soul led choices feel more authentic to you?

Clients may need a lot of support in this process. I cannot emphasise enough how hard it can be to make new heart and soul led choices and their ego will come along many times to challenge them during this process. The more aware and prepared they are, the stronger and more able they will feel to manage this when the ego appears. However, the benefits of living a more authentic life are so rewarding that this will give them the strength to keep going. Living mindfully is a significant part of this journey and will help them to deal with the bumps along the road and support them in stepping out of the Thought Bubble and egoic thinking. The more authentic you are as a therapist, the better the role model you will be to inspire and guide your clients. Practise what you preach!

Case examples

Below are some case examples to illustrate the different stages of HLP. The first case, Simon, will illustrate each of the stages of HLP. A few additional cases will then be described to illustrate the role of the observer and identify life lessons and gifts.

Case example of Simon

I introduced Simon in Chapter 3 when I was discussing the role of the ego. You may recall that he came to therapy a few years after experiencing a life-threatening illness that subsequently left him with anxiety symptoms. He had just left his wife of 26 years and was addicted to his business and work.

Simon was one of the youngest of six children growing up. His father worked hard, money was tight, and they lived in a council house. His dad had little involvement in their lives and his mother was the 'rock' although she was not tactile. Simon said he didn't feel like he was part of the family. He experienced some bullying throughout his schooling and was relieved when he left at 16 years old. Simon believed that he needed to achieve success financially and he managed to get a local job, which gave him a sense of feeling valued. He earned enough money to buy his parents' council home for them, although this caused more rifts with his siblings. Just when he had achieved a strong financial position he decided to give it all up and emigrate with his wife; this was at the same time that his wife found out she was pregnant with their first child. Simon had to start afresh, fighting for financial survival and he described this time as very tough. He said he suffered a nervous breakdown and felt absent during his wife's pregnancy. He worked all hours of the day to meet his commitments and reported that it was his pride that stopped him from coming back to the UK. A few years later his wife became pregnant again but miscarried at 20 weeks and this devastated him. Around the same time, Simon found himself broke, he had been promised a lot of money from his work that never materialised. This meant that he couldn't afford to come back to the UK. Money was so tight that he was struggling to afford food for his son and he asked his boss for a loan, which was given, but at a very high interest rate.

Simon managed to find another job, start earning again and could afford to buy a home. His wife had a few more miscarriages before giving birth to a daughter. Around this same time, he heard that his mother had died; this impacted him significantly and he described work as being the only tool that kept him going.

Financially, Simon's situation improved for one and a half years until the business he worked for started to have cash flow difficulties. He resigned because he didn't agree with the integrity of how the firm was being run. He then found himself back in the position of having nothing again and he was struggling to get out of bed in the morning. Simon's situation continued like this for the next 18 years; having money and then either losing it or changing jobs, which meant he had to start all over again. His wife had two more children (four in total) and she supported him throughout this time with every choice he made. They moved back to the UK in 2000 despite not being in a position to afford to do so. Again, the same patterns were repeated in his work.

Simon reported investing most of his time in work and found it hard to be physically and emotionally available for his family. In 2016, he suffered a pulmonary embolism and was told that he nearly died. The doctor at the time tried to explain how serious his condition was, but Simon didn't register the seriousness. He went back to work, again prioritising this over his own health and his family. After the pulmonary embolism, he started to experience anxiety symptoms that impacted on his ability to focus at work and it was his GP that suggested psychotherapy. When Simon came to see me, his relationship with his family had broken down and he had just moved out of the family home and was living in a hotel. His wife had clearly said to him 'You can live without me but not your work.'

Simon's challenges, traumas and attachment issues included:

- *Having a difficult relationship with his father and siblings and not feeling he belonged in his family, describing his relationship with his siblings as 'fractured.'*
- *Although he was close to his mother, there were no tactile interactions.*
- *He came from a financially deprived social background where there was little money, and this caused a strain on family relationships and behaviours.*
- *He was bullied at school.*
- *His wife experienced several miscarriages.*
- *He lost several jobs during his career.*

Simon's underlying blocks and restrictions were:

- *His sense of failure.*
- *Believing he was not good enough and not worthy. He felt ashamed of his family background.*
- *Not knowing his place within his family or work situations.*

Simon's repeated themes appeared to be:

- *His need to achieve financially to prove his self-worth.*
- *His struggle to hold on to money; each time he managed to start being successful he would change his circumstances and give everything up.*
- *Repeating his experience of his own deprivation of emotions from his childhood with his wife and children by disengaging at an emotional level, instead believing his sense of duty was to provide financially.*
- *Difficulty balancing work and family commitments.*
- *Several psychological breakdowns and most recently, anxiety.*

Becoming the observer

I tentatively brought in the role of Simon's ego at the end of the first session because I could identify how his pride was impacting on the decisions he had made and was continuing to make. Throughout all of our sessions I encouraged Simon to become the observer of his situations. As he learned to use this approach he was able to identify the role his ego played in how he had and was continuing to make decisions. It was possible for Simon to have conversations between his ego and his heart to assist him in starting to honour what his heart was trying to teach him. I taught Simon mindfulness so that he could become more aware, not just of his surroundings, but also of his situation when his ego was taking over and making the decisions. Guiding Simon to be the observer also enabled him to become the victor rather than take the victim role. He was learning to take full responsibility for his choices and actions and could start identifying how he had been in many challenges in order to experience and understand lessons throughout his life.

Life lessons

Simon was able to recognise a theme about learning to become vulnerable and that this was a theme that ran throughout his life and affected many areas including work, home, health and friendships. He was learning to recognise when to become vulnerable, when not to be vulnerable and when to allow others to be vulnerable. In his work, Simon recognised that he needed to be vulnerable and trust his colleagues to do a good job rather than feeling the constant need to do everything. His ego and pride had been stopping him from passing responsibility to others. Between him and his wife, he may have a joint lesson of partnership, learning to work together as a team rather than disjointedly. Simon recognised how he had allowed his wife to be subservient to him in the past but moving forward they could try to work together in true partnership.

Leap of faith and gifts

I had been working with Simon using the HASL model of HLP, as well as preparing him for some EMDR to work on his sense of failure in his past. During session seven, Simon recognised not only how his pride had affected major decisions in his life, but also how this had resulted in repeating patterns of behaviour where he would get stuck, which prevented him from learning important life lessons. Amazingly, after this session, Simon emailed me to say that he had returned to work and informed his staff that he was going to take some time off indefinitely. He was touched by the support and encouragement of his work colleagues. Simon was learning to let go of the hook that his ego had placed on work that was telling him that he was invaluable, indispensable and was needed to hold the company together. He was taking a leap of faith, having to trust that his staff were perfectly capable of doing their jobs and could manage without him. Simon also recognised that he didn't want to place any expectations on himself as to when or if he would return to work, nor any time frame by when he would make further decisions, as this would create more blocks and restrictions and minimise the chance of a successful outcome.

After Simon made this leap of faith he started focusing on his relationship with his wife. They agreed to meet up for dinner. His wife was understandably hesitant at first, because she was familiar with Simon saying the right thing but not being able to follow through with his intentions. However, they both persevered and started seeing each other most days; going out for day trips and family activities. Within a month, Simon reported that he had moved back into the family home. It was work in progress and he recognised that he needed to keep his momentum going and honour what his heart was guiding him to do, rather than being pulled back into repeated patterns and themes by his ego. We were able to process his early traumas relating to his sense of failure using EMDR.

Simon arrived one day for his appointment and discussed how he was inspired to create holiday accommodation opportunities for people who could not afford to go away. He also wanted to set up a free service with his wife to help others who didn't have the financial resources to set up a new business.

He said that this felt very important as part of his healing and spiritual journey. He wanted to give back to the universe and be of service to others. It was so wonderful to hear how he was 'awakening' and aligning with his authentic self. This demonstrates the power of the spiritual journey. Simon's gifts included freeing himself up from his addiction to work and starting to live a more authentic life which included helping others less fortunate than himself.

Other case examples

Thomas' life lessons

You may recall Thomas from Chapter 3, the gentleman in his 70s that came to see me believing he had 'severe depression.' It was several sessions into our work before an opportunity arose to introduce HLP to him. Thomas remained very stuck with not being able to let go of his successful business in order to retire. His history was not too dissimilar to Simon's, although he had come from a more fortunate financial background. He had been sent away to boarding school at eight years old and was deprived of love and affection from his parents and had huge expectations placed on him to be successful. At 73 years old he was still clinging on to his business, despite not feeling well enough or motivated to contribute because of his low mood. When I discussed the HL model he readily acknowledged the role of his ego and could identify how it was keeping him hooked into his work. I asked him to be an observer of his situation and wonder what this challenge was trying to help him learn and experience. He immediately said 'humility.' The spontaneity with which he replied suggested it resonated with him deeply and he felt that it was this that was keeping him stuck from making new choices and was relevant to his current psychological distress. We were then able to use his response to think about how he could make new informed heart led choices that embraced humility in order for him to find a more positive outcome and gain relief from his low mood.

Arjun's life lessons

I introduced Arjun in Chapters 2 and 5. During our second session we used the HASL model to two challenges that he had experienced during the week. I helped Arjun to recognise when his ego was talking to him and making him feel either the victim or the rescuer during confrontations with his wife.

I asked him to become the observer and look at each of the challenges sepa-rately to begin with, then reflect on what these opportunities were trying to help him understand or experience. With the first situation he felt that he was meant to be experiencing 'patience.' With the second challenge he believed this was trying to help him experience and understand 'assertiveness.' Inter-estingly, he then acknowledged that assertiveness was something he strug-gled with throughout his life and was probably why he didn't always make the most of opportunities. Assertiveness to Arjun was more likely to be a primary life lesson as he could see how it related to many challenges he had already encountered throughout his life: his upbringing and school, working career, first marriage and his current marriage. All by himself he identified how the life lesson worked in many ways, knowing when to be and when not to be assertive. In contrast, patience was more likely to be an everyday life lesson that he was currently encountering with the challenges at home.

Case example of everyday life lessons and gifts

Alice is a lady in her 30s whose situation is described in much more de-tail in Chapter 10. *Briefly, she had two very young children whom both had major health difficulties, one of which was life-threatening. We had already discussed HLP early on in therapy. During one session she felt inspired to share a recent event that demonstrated how she had acted as a teacher to a stranger in a brief encounter.*

Alice was in a taxi in London and the driver was very sociable. The driver was telling her how excited he was because his wife was expecting a baby af-ter six years of trying to conceive. Alice congratulated the man but was keen not to pursue the conversation too much because she didn't want to cause any worry to the driver due to her own children's health difficulties. How-ever, the taxi driver continued and asked Alice whether she had children. She told the man that she had two young children and that there had been some issues with conceiving but not nearly as long as his. The taxi driver wanted to ask her more about her children, so she was left with no option but to inform him that her children had major life-threatening health condi-tions, but that in spite of this she was grateful for their lives and cherished every moment. Alice told the man that while she wished she could take away her children's pain and suffering she wouldn't change what had happened because she now has a better appreciation of life and a gratitude that she had never felt before. The taxi driver was moved by her story and showed Alice a recording of his baby-to-be's heartbeat with such pride. He was so overwhelmed by Alice's story that he thanked her immensely and told her that he had been seeing himself as a victim because it had taken so long for his wife to conceive and he had been resenting his friends, whom he perceived had conceived children easily. Having listened to Alice's words he realised that he had a beautiful gift of appreciation for his forthcoming child that he hadn't understood before he met her. Rather than seeing himself as a victim he could observe the situation differently, with new eyes and aware-ness, which gave him such pride and gratitude; he told Alice no one had ever helped him to learn such appreciation before.

In this example, Alice could be considered a teacher to the taxi driver. Unknowingly and rather hesitantly to start with, she had engaged in a con-versation that had enabled another fellow being to be able to reflect differ-ently on their circumstances, switch from being the victim to the victor and receive the gift of gratitude and appreciation that would enable him to enjoy his child even more. The taxi driver had been learning through this process. A key point is that he was open to learning and Alice was open to teaching. Without this, so many opportunities get missed and people stay stuck in their own turmoil and distress.

Two final exercises are provided: the first encourages clients to re-write and re-frame their life story using HLP and the second exercise encourages clients to re-write and reframe their current life challenges using HLP. Both exercises are briefly described below but are available in more detail in the resource section.

Exercise 12

Re-writing one's life story using HLP

This exercise is found in the resource section. Clients are asked to re-write their life story so that they can reflect back on their journey so far. Using an HLP perspective they then have the opportunity to re-write and reframe their life story using the concepts already learned. These include:

1 Identifying their blocks and restrictions.
2 Identifying the repeated patterns in their life.
3 Understanding how challenges have occurred in order to experience life lessons.
4 Identifying reasons why they have had experiences or encounters with people to learn, teach or heal.
5 Identifying what the gifts are that they can now take away from these experiences.

Re-writing a story can be a very powerful way for clients to not only take ownership of their narrative, but to also reflect back and have a different perspective on the challenges they have experienced. This can increase their insight and awareness and hopefully guide them to make new choices moving forward in life rather than repeating themes.

Exercise 13

Re-writing current life challenges using HLP

This exercise, found in the resource section, can be introduced to your clients once you have explained HLP and how it relates to everyday life challenges, as well as the more significant challenges they have encountered. Re-writing current life challenges is an opportunity for clients to resolve issues more quickly, by identifying what opportunities these challenges are trying to provide them with so that they can make new informed choices. Using HLP, clients have the opportunity to re-write and reframe these current challenges using the concepts already learned, including understanding:

1 Everyday life lessons as well as their primary life lessons.
2 The reasons why they have had experiences or encounters with people to learn, teach or heal.
3 What the gifts are that they can now take away from these experiences?

Summary

- The aim of HLP is to provide clients with a technique to break out of the repetitive cycle that is maintaining their psychological distress.
- Clients are taught how to become the observer of their challenges so that they can assess the situation with a more detached perspective and identify their life lesson/s.
- Exploring the concept of life lessons can enable clients to make new informed choices rather than repeating previous familiar patterns of behaviour.
- Making new informed choices that are heart and soul led rather than ego led encourages clients to honour their authentic selves.
- Re-writing one's life story and current challenges using HLP may help increase clients' insight and awareness of their challenges and life lessons.

Heart and Soul Led model and soul level work

When you do things from your soul, you feel a river moving in you, a joy.

Rumi

Chapter 8 focuses on the additional components of the HASL model. It not only encourages clients to start living life through their heart and soul but also incorporates the option of soul level healing alongside the work you are already planning to carry out with your clients, where blocks and restrictions may have occurred at a soul level. Different ways in which these blocks and restrictions can be healed using soul therapies are also suggested. When I refer to soul therapies this often includes past life work. In addition, this chapter will provide an overview of some of the beliefs held about the origins of souls, including information about how souls work together in soul groups in order to support each other in their life lessons. An overview of karmic relationships will also be provided, illustrated with a case example.

Figure 8.1 illustrates the HASL model and additional key areas include:

- Soul level blocks and restrictions.
- Helping clients to move their awareness into their heart AND SOUL and start recognising what new choices they can make to move forward in their life.
- Supporting clients in achieving the gifts that they can take away from challenges that are heart AND SOUL led, based on making new choices. This may require clients to take leaps of faith.

Possible indications that soul level blocks and restrictions may be impacting on a client's life are where there are significant, toxic, or enmeshed relationship difficulties. This could be with another key person (typically someone in their family, a close friend, acquaintance, or work colleague), or it may be clear that your client has a major repeated issue with a certain aspect of their life, for example, finances, difficulty in conceiving children, or social, work, or systemic issues. Some therapists may have training in different soul level work or past life modalities and therefore may be comfortable including this in the package of care they offer their

DOI: 10.4324/9781003613749-11

Challenges, trauma and attachment difficulties from past lives

Blocks and restrictions at a soul level

Repeated patterns of behaviour or
situations during past lives

Current life challenges, trauma and
attachment difficulties

Current life blocks and restrictions

Current life repeated patterns of behaviour
or situations

EGO

Psychological distress

EGO

Becoming the observer

Soul therapies

Identify what life lessons can be experienced

EGO

HEART AND SOUL

Make same choices

Make new choices

Attain gifts

Self-love and authenticity

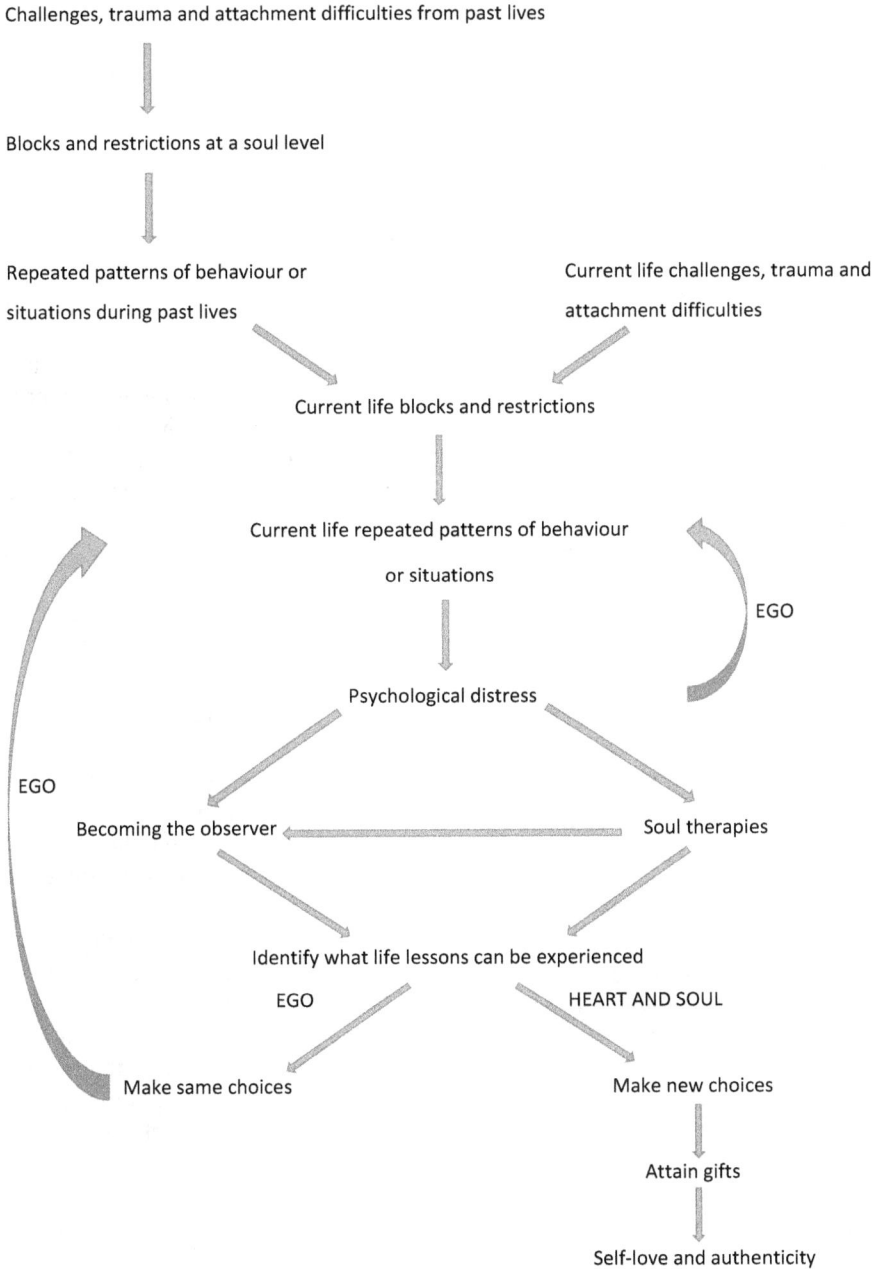

Figure 8.1 The Heart and Soul Led model

clients if clinically justified. For most, I would imagine that it is a topic you may raise with your clients, but then refer on to another practitioner who specialises in soul level work. If interested, I provide my clients with details of a spiritualist colleague of mine who is very skilled in soul therapies and in conjunction with this I keep focused on current life therapeutic work. Unless you are trained in offering soul therapies within your clinical practice, it is not your role to go into details with your client about what you believe may be their specific soul blocks and restrictions because you may well be wrong! Therefore, if you are even considering opening up this topic with your client, keep it as broad as possible, just opening up the discussion that there may be soul blocks and restrictions and then advise your client to seek further support if they wish to discover more.

Even if a client may have some soul blocks and restrictions, this doesn't mean that they need to undertake soul therapies. Sometimes just increasing your client's awareness of this area is enough to help them make new choices that are heart and soul led. Soul therapies may be beneficial when a client wants to make changes but is really struggling despite their best efforts, and it may be that the soul level blocks and restrictions are impacting on their ability to move forward. Clearing such blocks may help free them up and enable them to make the necessary new choices that are more authentic to them.

Origins of souls

There are different spiritual views and beliefs about where souls originated. Newton (2011) suggested that a soul belongs to a primary soul group or soul cluster and that this group works as a collective to facilitate each soul in experiencing their own individual life lessons. He believes that souls work together in order to LEARN, TEACH, and HEAL. Joint lessons can be part of this experience, but the main aim is to help each individual soul experience their primary (and secondary) life lesson. Some spiritual practitioners believe that our soul choses different incarnations in which to experience life lessons through different encounters and challenges, working with its primary soul group so that each soul is supporting each other. Before each incarnation, Weiss and Weiss (2012) proposed that souls choose with other souls (by making 'agreements' with each other) who will take the significant role as each of the main family members, for example, who will be the mother, father, siblings, and children. They suggest it is similar to creating a script for a drama and different souls from the primary soul group will decide which character they will play and the basis of the different scenes. During another incarnation the roles may be completely different, but the basic principle remains the same – each soul is provided with an opportunity to experience their own life lesson by learning, teaching and healing, as well as facilitating other souls. Other soul groups interact and facilitate each other during this process, which is why situations can happen in home life, work life, relationships etc. at the same time. In a particular lifetime, souls from another soul group may agree to help out by acting as a 'stand-in' or an 'extra part' to facilitate other souls' experience in their life lessons. Not every incarnation therefore is a major learning opportunity for each soul – some will have the lead roles or parts in the play or scene, but others will be 'extras.'

Joint lessons are believed to have been agreed between souls before an incarnation, or may be carried over from a previous incarnation if there is still some experience or learning that is felt beneficial to continue. Some clients will have fewer challenges to face during this lifetime, perhaps as a rest from a previous tough past life, or perhaps to facilitate others close to them to heal themselves. A soul may have agreed before incarnating to support others on their journey in this lifetime by playing a particular role in their lives but does not necessarily need to experience their own trauma or issues.

Introducing the idea of soul level blocks and restrictions

If your client is interested in spirituality and open to the presence of a soul and the idea of reincarnation, I would follow the same instructions detailed in Chapter 7, adapting it to the HASL model by using 'heart and soul' throughout the script. Once you have gone through this you can then introduce the idea of soul level blocks and restrictions. It is important to highlight to clients that this is based on certain spiritual beliefs and there is no scientific proof. I use the following description with my clients:

> There is a view that our souls are on a journey in order to experience a life lesson and that they may go through many different lifetimes in order to facilitate this process. What can happen during lifetimes is that we may find ourselves in difficult or challenging situations where we have been forced to do something against our wishes. An example is being forced to marry someone you didn't love, often for the preservation of family honour, or not being allowed to marry someone you loved, because you or your lover were not deemed to come from a good enough or worthy background. We may have been forced to fight in a war or battle even though this was against our values. There are many different scenarios, and this is what frequently happened in history – examples are illustrated in period dramas such as *Pride and Prejudice*. When these situations happened, and souls were forced to do something against their values, some believe that this created blocks and restrictions at a soul level. Ideas of such blocks and restrictions could include making vows of self-sacrifice, obedience, penitence, poverty, or chastity. Sometimes contracts were made between souls, for example, a healing, protection or soulmate contract. Other potential blocks and restrictions include pacts, bindings, and curses. The difficulty when such blocks and restrictions occurred is that these could possibly have been carried through to and impacted on subsequent lifetimes. This can make it even more challenging to learn life lessons or make choices in keeping with our authentic self.

At this stage, I would use the HASL model (Figure 8.1) to show how past life challenges may lead to soul level blocks and restrictions that create repeated patterns of behaviour during past lives (top left hand of the diagram). This then feeds into current life traumas which create current life blocks and restrictions. The other additional component of the HASL model is the option of undertaking soul therapy work to help clear soul level blocks and restrictions.

A typical question that your client may ask is:

So, how do I clear these soul blocks and restrictions?

At this stage, I would introduce the notion of soul therapies.

Soul therapies

There are several different soul therapies available that offer soul healing. These are all based on spiritual beliefs rather than facts and it is therefore impossible to prove the validity of such work. You are therefore requested to consider such information objectively and if interested, explore any areas that resonate with you. If you are interested in discussing some work with your clients, again it is imperative that you make clients aware that these are based on spiritual beliefs. You may have a particular interest in one area or know of colleagues who carry out this work. I have detailed below a few of these that I am familiar with and recommend, but please don't assume this is exhaustive. Work within your field of expertise and knowledge and, if in doubt, recommend that your client explore for themselves what feels right to them, making sure they go to someone who is reputable.

The Akashic Records

The Hungarian philosopher, Ervin Laszlo, who was an advocate of quantum consciousness, wrote about how he believed the Akashic Field represents an energy and information-carrying field that contains knowledge about all the universes, past and present (Laszlo, 2007). Howe (2010, p. 3) suggested that the Akashic Records is a 'dimension of consciousness that contains a vibrational record of every soul and its journey.' In other words it is believed to represent a library of information that is held in the fifth dimension (whereas we reside in the third dimension) and which contains all the knowledge and information about each soul's journey through every incarnation. O'Malley (2018) suggested that the eighth chakra (situated 20 cm above the head) can access the Akashic Records with the main function being to connect the physical body to a higher energy source. There are various spiritual practitioners who have developed soul level healing and training packages that incorporate working with the Akashic Records. For example, Andrea Hess developed a Soul Realignment programme, (www.soulrealignment.com), Steve Nobel developed his own 121 Soul Matrix healing package (www.thesoulmatrix.com) and

Liz King (www.liz-king.co.uk) offers Akashic Record clearing and training in addition to other soul therapies.

Within the Akashic Records, as well as other soul therapies, it is believed that there are a number of different blocks and restrictions that can arise from traumas and challenges at a soul level, including:

- Vows, for example, self-sacrifice, obedience, penitence, chastity, poverty, and suffering.
- Contracts, for example, soulmate, healing, and protection.
- Spells, curses, pacts, and bindings.
- Anger spears and negative thought forms (in the Akashic Records these are believed to only happen in present life and are not carried through different incarnations).

It is proposed that such blocks and restrictions can cause damage to the chakras, tares to the Golden Web (believed to be an energetic membrane that surrounds an individual's energy body in order to keep the energetic being whole and integrated), Godspark damage (it is thought that within our hearts there is an energy flame or spark that is representative of the Divine within us and this is fed through an energy line that runs from the Divine Source) and soul facet loss.

The process of the Akashic Record healing

As mentioned above, the Akashic Records are believed to be held in the fifth dimension, existing on an etheric level rather than a physical third-dimensional level. It is often referred to as a 'library' or 'Book of Life,' containing every soul's pathway ever taken, including all past life memories and experiences and blocks and restrictions. It is imperative that any client embarking on this work gives their permission for their Akashic Records to be read rather than feel they are being cajoled into undertaking this healing. It is believed (and reiterated during the training) that it is impossible to access someone's Akashic Records without their permission or higher purpose. The information will just be blocked by their soul and the Divine Source. It is therefore trusting or having the faith that the soul must agree and if it does not want to embark on this work, it just won't happen!

I can refer to the process used by my colleague, Liz King, who is highly experienced in working with the Akashic Records. Before meeting a client, Liz will carry out a 'distant reading' (in other words spiritually connect to the client's Akashic Records in the client's absence), which usually takes a few hours where she identifies their overall soul profile and the blocks and restrictions and the story behind what caused any blocks and restrictions. Liz then arranges a session with the client, usually lasting 90 minutes to feed back this information. During this session Liz will ask the client whether the information resonates with them and will ask for examples of this based on the client's current lifetime experiences – she won't just take their word for it! As with any therapy or healing we participate in, it has to make sense to the client, otherwise there is no benefit for anyone. This is why it is important that you only recommend practitioners who are reputable and authentic. Finally, once the session is finished, Liz will complete the work by re-accessing the client's Akashic Records and clearing the blocks and restrictions identified. The client is then given a customised 21-day prayer (which is very angelic and non-denominational) that helps filter the information through to their everyday awareness and consciousness and confirms their wish to have their soul blocks and restrictions cleared. Akashic Record healing is gaining in popularity which unfortunately means that there are some 'healers' who are monopolising on this and charging excessive amounts of money and not providing accurate or comprehensive readings, so please do take time to make sure the person you decide to work with is authentic and credible.

If a client expresses interest in finding out about healing at a soul level, I intro-duce the topic of the Akashic Records as a possible way of facilitating the clearing of soul level blocks and restrictions. I have undertaken some training in the Akashic Records as well as had a lot of healing using this modality, so I am comfortable discussing this notion with clients. If your client shows a sense of curiousness and openness to the idea of the Akashic Records, then it is usually safe to still introduce this work and let them reflect on whether this resonates with them over time and to carry out their own research. The important thing is not to push your client into any work that doesn't feel comfortable for them. If you have experience in other soul therapies, then you may prefer to talk about these with your clients instead or just keep the topic of soul level work very open and allow your clients to explore for themselves if they so choose.

This is how I introduce the topic of Akashic Records:

There is some spiritual work that can be done to help identify which blocks and restrictions your soul is carrying and then clear these so that you are freer to make new choices moving forward. It is a healing using the Akashic Records, which is ultimately a form of soul therapy. In essence, we live in the third di-mension, and the Akashic Records is metaphorically like a library in the fifth dimension (etheric level) and contains all of the information about everyone's soul. It is believed that accessing this information, with your permission, by someone trained to work using the Akashic Records, not only can provide you with knowledge of your soul's origin, but also identify any blocks and restric-tions at a soul level during specific past lives including what the actual story was that created these initial blocks. Once the information has been accessed, you will be given this knowledge and made sure that it resonates with you and your own current life experiences. Following this, the soul blocks and restrictions will be cleared in your Akashic Records on your behalf. You will then receive a 21-day prayer, which is very angelic and non-denominational, to facilitate the clearing and strengthening of this knowledge from your higher self into your everyday conscious awareness. You are then free to make new choices in life, if you so wish, without these blocks in place.

Working using the Akashic Records is often like peeling an onion; sometimes you will only need to do a small amount of clearing in order to make a significant difference in your life, sometimes further work is required, depending on what challenges you have had in the past. Initially it is advisable to have your own soul blocks and restrictions cleared first. It is then possible to do some overlays in which you can clear on your side the blocks and restrictions between you and someone else with whom you have a very difficult, challenging or significant relationship in this lifetime. Difficult relationships are often believed to be a replay of challenges you have had with them in past lives. Clearing the blocks and restrictions on your side will not only help you understand the dynamics better but will also free you up to make new choices on how to manage the relationship moving forward.

It is possible for a parent or carer to clear their children's Akashic Records on their behalf, up to the point at which their child becomes 18 years old. Generally the child is unaware of this because they may not have the level of spiritual insightfulness, or maturity to recognise the benefits of this work themselves. If someone chooses to have more than one Akashic Record clearing completed, either on their own individual Akashic Records, or as an overlay with another person's Akashic Records, they are likely to be told about their primary and secondary life lessons as well as any joint lessons with that specific person. This is not usually provided during the first appointment given the volume of information that they will be told about their soul (soul profile and place of origination) as well as their main blocks and restrictions. Despite having some training using the Akashic Record, this is not a service I offer my clients. One of the reasons is that I like to maintain some professional boundaries, especially where clients have been referred via insurance companies. At the moment, I believe that I am a catalyst for opening up the topic of spirituality with clients and that it is my role to guide and support them with the beginning part of this journey. I can then direct my clients to other trained spiritual practitioners if they wish to discover more for themselves and I can then continue to support them psychologically. However, if the Akashic Records is of interest to you and you would like to offer this as part of your service to clients, then it is definitely worth considering accessing the training. Otherwise, try to make links with someone who can offer this therapy. I am fortunate that I have a spiritual colleague who works purely in spiritual healing and I provide my clients with her details if they are keen to pursue this. She is able to offer Akashic Record readings, soul retrieval work, shamanic work, past life regression, psychic readings, hypnosis and many other healing therapies. Many of my clients have reported that this joint working has very beneficial and some case examples will be discussed in Chapter 10.

While this may be a new area to you, all I can encourage you to do is to try and keep an open mind and don't judge or form opinions based on ignorance. Most of my clients hold a sense of curiosity and once they have embarked on this healing, they are completely blown away by what they discover and the parallels to their experiences in their current lifetime. I have never had a client be disappointed or disagree with what they have discovered so far. However, never force or over-encourage a client to complete this work – they must only do this if it feels right to them and is at the right time in their life.

Shamanic journeying and soul retrieval

A number of psychotherapists have incorporated soul retrieval and shamanic jour-neying into their practice, for example, Alberto Villoldo (2005) and Sandra Inger-man (2014). Sandra Ingerman talks about Shamanism as a pathway to opening up and learning to live life through one's heart, ideas in keeping with HLP. Irene Siegel (2017, 2018) has written about how she integrates her shamanic practice into her clinical work, which includes her EMDR practice, therefore adopting a BioPsychoSocioSpiritual approach similar to mine.

Shamanic journeying involves the use of rhythm, often through drumming, as this is believed to help individuals enter an altered state of consciousness so that they connect with the spiritual dimension of reality. The word shaman comes from the Siberian Tungusic word for a spiritual leader or 'one who is raised' and this title can often be interchanged with medicine man/woman or healer. Shamans believe that there are three worlds: the Middle World, which is where we physically exist, work and have relationships and the Lower and Upper Worlds, which are not physi-cal places, but archetypal and energetic realms that are not bound by time. The Lower World is the realm of the soul and contains all information on our soul's his-tory, in other words our past. The Upper World is the realm of our destiny and our spirit and travelling to this world can help us access our destiny and life purpose. Working with an experienced shaman, it is believed that a person can enter the Lower and Upper Worlds to discover information that may assist them in making sense of their lives. Travelling to the Lower World can also help people to retrieve missing parts of their soul that may have been lost through past traumas.

Past life regression

The aim of regression therapy is to heal mental, physical, and spiritual issues by identifying, reliving, and resolving past traumas. It is based on the belief that past life traumas are held in our etheric, mental and physical energy fields (Tomlinson, 2012). These traumas may have occurred in this lifetime or past lifetimes. The process typically involves using hypnosis to get the client into an altered state of consciousness so that they can 'bridge back' and reconnect with the original trauma. Once connected, clients can gain a greater understanding of what the situa-tion was that caused the trauma and find ways to process and heal the trauma. Often this involves forgiveness, either to the person who caused the trauma, or perhaps to the recipient of the trauma.

Soul readings

A close friend of mine went to see a practitioner who offered soul readings. Information from soul readings may provide an understanding of a person's life at a soul level, consider the individual's soul journey including past lives as well as an explanation of the challenges and relationships that have been encountered in this life, their meanings and purpose. My friend had experienced a difficult relationship with her father while he was alive. She had also never managed to conceive. This is my friend's recount of her soul level reading, which links into the idea discussed at the beginning of the chapter that souls contract with each other before each incarnation in order to help heal, teach, or learn from each other.

It was explained that my husband contracted before this lifetime to help me explore my spirituality and that in order to facilitate that, he would provide for me materially. He was injured in a previous life and couldn't work, so now he wishes to work a lot in this lifetime. He also contracted to help me heal my relationship with men in this lifetime, as I have had many lifetimes of being abused by men and trapped in relationships. For example, I was trapped in marriages with abusive partners where I could not leave and stayed for the children.

My Dad came through in the reading and apologised to me. He feels that he could have done more to help. He said that he deeply regretted not being a better father and was unable to demonstrate love in the usual way. He said he wished that he could have held my hands, looked me in the eyes, and said 'I love you,' but he couldn't. He was like a caged animal – emotionally vulnerable but pretended not to be. I contracted to come into my Dad's life as his daughter to heal him. I felt that he could not resist loving a beautiful baby and would feel that love through his soul. The reality was that I was deeply affected by his anger, even in my cot, and it left me unsure of what to expect. I carry this pattern through into my relationship with my husband. If he feels unhappy or angry then I worry and cannot settle, but there is no need for me to do that.

During this lifetime I am free from children to allow 'space' and to heal old wounds. There was a possibility of children in this lifetime, but it was a path not followed and that's fine. My Dad came through holding a baby boy lost by someone in the family and said that healing of the family is very helpful for him. This seemed to highlight for me the importance of healing the ancestors, those who have gone before. I now wonder if that baby was the child I could have had but didn't and by not following the pathway of being a mother again have I been able to offer some deep healing for myself in this lifetime, and also has it helped to heal the family as a whole.

This soul reading helped my friend to understand more fully the relationships in her life, find a place of peace from the difficulties she had experienced with her father and also realise why she hadn't managed to have children in this lifetime.

Other spiritual healing techniques

There are many alternative or spiritual therapies that are available depending on one's own belief system and it is beyond the bounds of this book to go into detail of such therapies. They include Angelic Reiki, traditional Reiki, Diamond Approach, working with crystals, chakra clearing, yoga, various types of massage, acupuncture, reflexology, herbalism, and homoeopathy to name but a few. I have met a number of alternative practitioners who also work at a past life level, including reflexologists, acupuncturists, and homoeopaths. If your clients are interested in alternative therapies, the key is that they find someone they can trust because, as with any type of practitioner, therapist or healer, some are wonderful and incredibly talented, and others perhaps do not quite reach the level required to offer a good and effective service. In addition, there are other resources available to clients; either reading materials or oracle cards, mediation exercises etc. Wayne Dyer has written many spiritual books to guide and inspire individuals to embrace a loving life by being kind, generous, thoughtful, caring and patient with fellow citizens and be a true vessel of unconditional love from the Divine Source.

Karma

Discussing karma is probably the most controversial aspect of this book. So many of us prefer to avoid the concept of karma, let alone discuss what it could represent or mean to us. When we think of karma, most people think they must have done something terribly wrong to explain their suffering or discomfort. For example, if they have an illness or condition, or find themselves in tough circumstances, they may blame this on karma and say that they have obviously done something awful in a past life. This view is not a fair representation of karma and can lead to confusion and misunderstandings.

Different religions and belief systems have various interpretations of karma, which of course makes the whole topic very confusing. The Sanskrit interpretation of karma is based on action, work or deed, as well as cause and effect, where the intentions of an individual (cause) have a bearing on the future of that individual (effect). It distinguishes between good and bad karma. Thus if someone has performed good deeds in their life this will result in good karma. On the other hand, if an individual has had the intent of causing bad or harmful deeds in life then this will lead to future suffering. In her book showing how a person can access their own Akashic Records, Linda Howe (2010) discussed how reincarnation is not about seeing lifetimes as 'good' or 'bad,' and karma is not about 'reward' or 'punishment.' Tomlinson (2012) explained karma as a way of experiencing both sides of a situation and how this may be carried over various lifetimes to facilitate greater understanding and development.

In Akashic Record training, karma is differentiated between 'negative unjustified karma' and 'negative karma.' It is believed that negative unjustified karma occurs during a situation where a soul has been forced to do something against its wishes, or that goes against its Divine purpose. For example, if someone was forced to marry another person for money rather than for love or prevented from doing a job that they had their heart set on. They may have been in love with someone, but because it wasn't in agreement with what their family expected, they were prevented from being with that person.

In contrast, negative karma is believed to occur between two or more souls. If someone has consciously killed or been very instrumental in the death of another individual, then it is believed that this creates negative karma at a soul level, because this action goes against the Divine Source. Therefore the soul who was instrumental in someone else's death would be considered the 'bearer' of the karma and the soul who died would be the 'recipient' of the karma. In subsequent reincarnations the bearer and recipient souls are likely to enter into another situation or relationship to provide an opportunity for the negative karma to be healed. The way to heal negative karma and break the pattern is to learn to approach the situation differently. This requires the 'recipient' to operate with an open, loving and compassionate heart to show forgiveness to the 'bearer,' while also teaching them through love and compassion to take responsibility for their wrong-doing.

Negative karma is the only block or restriction that cannot be cleared using the Akashic Records. In a similar way to how Tomlinson (2012) described using past life regression, it is believed that the only way negative karma can be cleared is for the recipient to teach or heal the bearer about true forgiveness and support them in aligning with a more positive loving way of living through unconditional love. Negative karmic relationships are very challenging and may present themselves in abusive or toxic relationships. The difficulty is that the soul bearer of the negative karma usually lacks the insight that they have done anything wrong and tends to blame the soul of the recipient for any difficulties. The recipient typically encounters abusive or destructive behaviour from the bearer and often becomes the victim over and over again. Thus these relationships end up in vicious repeated patterns of behaviour. Negative karma can be healed when the recipient learns to step outside of the fearful victim role and take a different approach. This usually involves the recipient putting up protective boundaries but keeping their heart and soul open with Divine or unconditional love, forgiving the bearer and holding on to the hope that the bearer will become a kinder, more loving and compassionate person.

Case study illustrating karma

Franky was a 15-year-old who came to see me because of suicidal thoughts, self-harm, anger, and relationship difficulties, especially with her dad. Initially she engaged really well, but unfortunately she then got into a relationship with a teenage boy. Franky's behaviour then deteriorated significantly to the extent that she dropped out of school and her behaviour at home became so problematic that social services became involved. Franky would take vengeance out on her mother both verbally and physically and she decided to leave home. This was highly problematic because of her age, but Franky refused to live with her parents. She also disengaged from our work. CAMHS became involved, but Franky would not attend sessions with them either, so social services became the main overseers of her care. I continued to support her mother, Tina, who was a very gentle and caring lady and highly concerned about her daughter. Tina was very open to spirituality and the concept of a soul, so we discussed the HASL model and she readily engaged with the Akashic Record work with my colleague, not only having her Akashic Records cleared, but also Franky's and an overlay between them (lifetimes that they have shared together).

An overlay of both Tina's and Franky's Akashic Records was carried out by my spiritual colleague, Liz King. The process of this has been explained earlier in the chapter. Liz would have known very little about Tina or Franky before completing this work (except their birth name, date of birth, and place of birth), which in many ways is important so that she is not influenced by their stories. Before attending the session, Liz would have accessed their Akashic Records in the fifth dimension, identified the original lifetime where any soul blocks and restrictions occurred between Franky and Tina and found out the story behind such difficulties. Tina then had a session with Liz to discover what had been found in her Akashic Records before Liz cleared the soul blocks and restrictions for them both.

The information has been voluntarily provided to me by Tina who reported that it resonated with her own spiritual beliefs and her current lifetime circumstances with her daughter. There is no scientific proof or evidence to support or verify any of the Akashic Record information reported and it is based on spiritual beliefs rather than facts. However, it is important that you make your own conclusion on the information provided in an objective way. During the session with Liz, Tina was told that the main blocks and restrictions included negative karma. Tina later reported to me that the overlay increased her understanding of her challenging relationship with Franky, which helped her to find some relief and detachment from the emotional difficulties she experienced with her daughter and gave her the strength to work at healing the negative karma.

It was around the time of the Tudor Court in the 1500s when HRH Queen Elizabeth I was reigning. Tina was incarnated as a female and Franky as a male and they were siblings in this lifetime. Their family lived in court, as their parents had been serving faithfully as courtiers for years. The son (Franky) got involved with the wrong crowd who were trying to discredit the Queen. The son was very popular but easily influenced and led astray. It soon became known that the son was working with others against the court. His father wanted to warn him, but his mother secretly agreed with what her son was doing. His sister (Tina) warned him not to be so vocal, but he took offence against her. The sister then told someone in authority with the hope that they would be able to influence and protect her brother, but unfortunately this didn't work out as planned. The son was arrested and taken to the Tower along with others in his group. He was given the opportunity for clemency if he gave information about their plans, but he refused and was later hanged, and his head was left on a spike for all to see. The brother was very angry with his sister and wanted revenge before his death and so arranged for her to be murdered.

If the brother had not arranged for his sister's death, there would have been unjustified negative karma between them because the sister had been trying to help protect her brother, but unfortunately it had backfired and resulted in her brother's death. However, given that he instigated his sister's murder, negative karma was created, with the brother (Franky) being the bearer and the sister (Tina) being the recipient.

Tina was told that she had shared seven lifetimes with Franky: four as siblings, two as parent/child and one as friends. They have a joint lesson of integrity. Tina's primary life lesson is empowerment and Franky's is compassion. Tina is therefore trying to teach Franky integrity but also needs to remain empowered in the challenges and abuse she experiences. Franky is experiencing challenges to help experience compassion as well as integrity through her mother. Tina's role is also to try to heal the negative karma by both keeping an open heart while maintaining some protective boundaries; incredibly difficult to do when a relationship is so hurtful, abusive and relentless.

Summary

- The HASL model considers the option of soul blocks and restrictions.
- If your client is not comfortable with the notion of past lives but believes in the concept of a soul, you can still use the HASL, just omit reference to past life traumas and soul healing. You may find it easier instead to use the HL model in such instances, referring to 'heart and soul' instead of 'heart.'
- Some spiritual therapies believe that soul level blocks and restrictions can occur from current or past life traumas.

- Some spiritual beliefs include the notion that souls belong to a primary soul group and together work as a collective to support each other in learning, teaching and healing, to enable the progression of their individual life lessons.
- Different soul groups can work together to provide additional support as required.
- There are different types of soul therapies, including Akashic Records, soul retrieval work and past life regression.
- The Akashic Records is believed to hold all the information of a soul's journey throughout its lifetimes and contains the knowledge of all life blocks and restrictions at a soul level. Working with a practitioner trained in accessing the Akashic Records can provide your client with the knowledge underlying their blocks and restrictions and enable them to clear these at a soul level.
- Clearing soul blocks and restrictions can facilitate your client to make new choices at a soul level rather than repeating recurrent themes. However, this is now a conscious choice on how they live their life – they may still decide to repeat themes even though the blocks and restrictions have been removed.
- It is believed that negative karma is the only block that cannot be cleared using the Akashic Records or past life therapies. The importance of negative karma is that resolution and forgiveness is achieved during a lifetime between souls concerned in order to heal this karma.

9

HLP and beyond

It is during the darkest moments that we must focus to see the light.

Aristotle

The aim of this chapter is to reflect on a range of different topics that extend beyond the actual HLP models. This starts with a review of the benefits of using HLP with clients, but also considers occasions when it may not be suitable to use HLP. How to recognise something positive out of every challenge is then discussed. This will be followed by details of various physical and emotional symptoms that some of your clients may experience during their spiritual journey. It is important to be aware of such possible symptoms so that you and your clients can be prepared to manage them appropriately. Next, as with any type of therapy we offer, it is essential that clinicians take care of themselves in all areas of their lives, and some ideas are provided which can be used in addition to mindfulness, as well as using HLP in your own life. HLP can also be used in a supervisory context and this will be discussed briefly.

What are the benefits of using HLP?

Using HLP is a process that some clients will readily engage with and understand, but others may need more support and practise. While it may sometimes be obvious to you what the answers are, it is far more powerful when clients can become the observer and increase their awareness to find their own answers. Teaching this process to clients can facilitate both their learning and their practice of this skill so that they can adopt a similar perspective when future challenges arise. Some of the benefits I have observed clinically include clients:

- Learning to become the observer and gain a broader understanding of challenges more quickly.
- Stop seeing themselves as a victim but rather as a victor.
- Spending less time in challenges and therefore experience less psychological distress.

DOI: 10.4324/9781003613749-12

- Recognising how challenges are opportunities to experience life lessons.
- Start moving away from their ego and begin to make new choices that honour their heart and soul.
- Becoming more aligned with their authentic self.

I have used HLP with both adults and teenagers. It is important to remember that when working with adolescents, they can be easily influenced as their brain and identity are still developing. We need to support them in finding their own truth and perspective, meeting them where they are at while recognising that this may change during the course of the time you work with them. Younger children are less likely to be able to grasp some of the ideas because they may not have developed sufficient cognitive skills to master the key concepts. However, I do believe that they can still reap the benefits if some areas of this work are completed with their parents who can act as excellent role models for their children.

Are there times when HLP is not appropriate?

As with any of the work we offer, it is important to reflect on the reasons why we introduce a therapy or a particular way of working with clients. I don't believe in fitting clients into boxes, but instead in finding the right approach for them that is tailored to their needs and requirements. This also applies when considering using HLP with clients. There is no harm at all in asking about a person's spiritual beliefs, so long as you as a therapist are respectful and open and work with your client's belief system without imposing your own views.

I believe HLP can be utilised with any client who is open-minded, motivated, and has a level of psychological insight. Working with this model does touch on some sensitive areas where there may be resistance, in particular discussing their ego. However, if this is done in an empathic manner where the ego is explained as their over-thinking, over-analysis, or self-image, the client will usually grasp this concept openly and be willing to acknowledge the power their ego has on their life. The other area where there may be some resistance is in discussing the role of the victim. Encouraging your client to learn to step out of a situation and become an observer can be very empowering and can help them to reflect more clearly on the situation, make wiser decisions, and have a better understanding of what they can learn as a person. I have actually been pleasantly surprised that my clients have not taken offence when discussing either the ego or the victim role. In fact, on the contrary, they show relief and understanding to these ideas, especially as I am able to normalise them.

If your client is actively suicidal, psychotic, or highly dissociative, then obviously stabilisation must take priority. Risk management has to take precedence, as with any other therapy or intervention offered. Once all risks have been managed appropriately and your client is more stable and able to engage in a therapeutic way, then it is probably safe to introduce HLP. It may not always be suitable for some clients who have fragile complex personalities including traits or a diagnosis of certain personality disorder as they may not have developed the cognitive strength to understand or apply aspects of HLP.

Undertaking any soul level work using soul therapies also requires that your client is stable and not actively at risk or psychotic or unstable. Soul therapies can be very powerful so your client must be in a position where they can manage and cope with such changes as they are happening. Therefore making your client aware of the power of such interventions to be able to manage these appropriately is essential. Any therapist who offers soul therapies should also take this into consideration. When soul therapies are being used in addition to your therapeutic work it is imperative to work collaboratively with the other practitioner and discuss the timings of any planned intervention so that you are not overloading your client with too much at any given time.

Turning challenges into something positive

Many people experience great challenges and difficulties in their lives. The aim of HLP is to move them away from assuming the victim role where their ego is in charge. Instead of thinking 'Why is this happening to me?' perhaps a more helpful way would be to think 'Why shouldn't this be happening to me,' or 'What can I learn or understand from this experience?' The rate of cancer is on the increase, as are many other physical and emotional difficulties, so the likelihood of us experiencing something challenging, whether it is physical, emotional, mental, or spiritual is much more likely nowadays. If we find ourselves in tough circumstances, it doesn't mean we have done something wrong or need to be punished. It is a chance to learn and grow from the experience. When we learn to embrace such challenges rather than fight them, the experience can be much more fruitful and powerful and less stressful.

There are many examples of individuals who have undergone such inspirational journeys. Every week when I read the newspaper there are stories of individuals who have experienced various traumas and challenges, but who have turned their lives around and have turned this experience into something positive and wonderful to show that anything is possible if we allow and open up to the possibilities. Gandhi was an example of how to fight for civil rights using non-violent protest despite experiencing great resistance at a global level. Nelson Mandela spent years in prison campaigning to end Apartheid, putting his own needs aside to bring about positive change in society and there are many more examples throughout history. Stephen Hawking was another inspirational person. A renowned physicist and cosmologist, his motor neurone disease greatly impacted on his physical life, yet, despite this, he continued to educate the world with his wisdom and knowledge in a way that is far beyond what most of us could ever achieve. He died at the age of 76 which is pretty incredible given that when he was 22 years old he was told that he only had two years to live. Some people are debating whether he was the incarnation of Einstein, given the similarities in their wisdom and what they both achieved. Einstein was interestingly born on the same day that Stephen Hawking died, just 139 years earlier!

Such individuals were able, at times, to put their own needs and desires aside and endure incredible hardship for the benefit of the good of humanity. They encountered great resistance along the way, but this never deterred them from their mission and they succeeded.

Awakening symptoms

If your client chooses to embark on a spiritual journey, especially at a soul level, they may notice various symptoms at a physical, emotional, cognitive and etheric level. It is helpful for you or your clients to be aware of such symptoms while their body adjusts to the changes that are happening. These can include:

- **Increased sensitivity and awareness**. Your client may notice changes in their tastes such as with food and drink, including alcohol. What used to appeal to them may no longer be desirable, including fatty foods, meats and sugary foods. This may be the way their body is helping them to avoid foods and substances that are no longer required or will not benefit them moving forward. Your client may also become more aware of their surroundings and live more mindfully, finding beauty and appreciation that had previously gone unnoticed.
- **Physical changes**. Your client may find they have an increase in aches and pains in their bodies, especially around their head, neck and shoulders. Practising yoga or stretching can help as their bodies adjust to their increased spiritual awakening.
- **Mood changes**. As your client becomes more awakened, they may find themselves going through periods of low mood, anxiety, or anger as they rid themselves of past traumas – this is thought to be a natural part of the healing process (Dura-Vila, 2016). Encourage your client to mindfully embrace such changes and help them to understand that this is part of their healing, an opportunity to let go of past burdens and traumas. Some clients who really embrace their spiritual journey may find themselves in the 'Dark Night of the Soul' (Moore, 2011). In addition, your client may also start to feel more grace, joy and bliss as they increase their awareness.
- **Energy changes**. Your client may find themselves absolutely exhausted at times for no apparent reason or buzzing with excess energy. This can fluctuate on a daily basis with no obvious pattern. Try to encourage your client to listen and work with what their body is trying to teach them, understanding what is happening in the here and now rather than forcing it to do something when they are not in the right energetic place.
- **Sleep issues**. A very common awakening symptom is changes in sleep patterns. Your client may go through phases where they are really struggling to sleep, perhaps waking up regularly or feeling very hot in the night. Other times they may notice that they need to sleep much more than usual. They may notice changes in their dreams, which can become more vivid. Offering some reassurance can help your client to not panic and also know that it is not long-lasting

and that things will return to an equilibrium with time. Encourage them to not fight this process and be gentler with themselves when sleep is affected, so that they do not burn themselves out, but instead embrace and work with these changes.

- **Changes in relationships and friendships.** As your client becomes more awakened they may notice a change in their feelings toward some friendships and relationships. This can be a difficult time, as your client may feel sad about such losses. However, they may notice that what used to be appealing in some relationships is no longer there, interests have changed. This isn't a bad thing, just hard to adjust to, as it is another way of letting go and moving forward to their more authentic selves. Clinging on to relationships that are no longer serving a purpose may hold your client back on their spiritual journey. Encourage them to have the faith and knowledge that this is a natural part of the healing journey and that new relationships will enter their lives that are more authentic and rewarding to them.
- **Feeling lost or alone.** Your clients may take a while to adjust to all the changes that are happening to them and at times feel very isolated and disconnected from their lives and people around them. They may feel abandoned, alone or misunderstood, or feel that no one understands what they are going through. It is therefore very important to offer a space for your clients to express themselves where they don't feel judged or criticised.

Your clients may experience none, some, or all of the above at any stage. I can relate to having experienced all of the above symptoms at different stages throughout my spiritual journey so far. Over the past few years my tastes in foods have changed, as have my relationships and interests. I have experienced extreme exhaustion, insomnia, and many, many sleepless nights where I was so hot that it felt like I was on fire. At one stage I had some tests done with my GP only to discover that I was in good health. Coming to some understanding and acceptance that I was possibly having energy shifts helped me to learn to relax and not fight the awakening symptoms, so that I could just accept them and be gentler to myself during these stages, particularly when I was tired. Embarking on a spiritual journey can be very lonely and frightening at times, but part of this journey is to recognise that when we attach or hook ourselves into situations or people it stops us from learning that we have everything we need within us. Finding a place of self-love and compassion is the ultimate goal of becoming aligned with the Divine Source and becoming our true authentic self.

Looking after yourself as a therapist

It is so important that you look after yourself as a therapist and become a good role model for your clients, regardless of whether you are on your own spiritual journey or not. I have already highlighted some of the awakening symptoms that can occur not only with your clients but also with yourself.

I live my life now through HLP; I have to practice what I preach! I have a good understanding of what I believe my life lessons are and I am much more mindful of challenges and recognise these as opportunities to continue to understand and experience key themes in my spiritual journey. I have to work at this every day and not take anything for granted. Sometimes this is easier said than done, but as I continue to do this I have noticed I live a more authentic life, which is easier and more graceful. That isn't to say it is a smooth ride, because it certainly isn't at times, but as my awareness and understanding improves, so does my resilience to manage challenges. In addition to using HLP, I engage in approximately two to three hours of self-care each day. This may sound decadent or impossible to some, but when I told myself that it was the most essential part of my day and enabled me to work at an energetic frequency that I aspire to (it's just that I wasn't getting paid during this time!), I somehow managed to build this into my daily routine. I also have to look after my body by taking care of what I eat and drink, meditating, taking regular exercise including cycling, walking and yoga, hobbies and interests, getting outside to connect with daylight and nature, and spending time with my family and special friends too. It is worth identifying which areas in your life nurture or enrich you and which areas are more draining and need changing.

As you start embracing spirituality into your life it is also sensible to look after yourself and your working environment. Ideas to look after yourself include:

1 Imagining yourself in a protective bubble which only allows positive energy through. Any negative energy is sent back into the universe to be cleared and cleansed.
2 Grounding yourself regularly. You can do this by being mindful, and really connecting with the environment around you. You can also imagine roots coming from your feet into the ground below, making you feel strong and secure and connected to the earth's energy.
3 Having regular Dead Sea salt baths may help decrease stress and remove any negative energy that you may be carrying within your energy field.
4 Meditation. This increases your capacity to contain not only your own spiritual journey, but also your capacity to contain your clients and the difficulties they are working through.
5 If you believe in a soul then you may find it helpful to connect to universal and Divine support, which, depending on your own beliefs, may include your own personal team of guides, teachers, angels, archangels, and so forth.

Ideas to look after your environment that may be considered beneficial depending on your beliefs include:

1 Clearing the energy space regularly either by smudging with sage or a smudge stick.
2 Using chimes or other sound healing, e.g. a singing bowl to cleanse the energy.

3 Using crystals to help keep the energy in the room at a positive vibration. Remember to cleanse these regularly.
4 Making sure there is regular fresh air that can flow through your environmental space to clear out negative or stale energies.

There are many more, some of which I have discussed elsewhere in more detail (Dent, 2025) so don't just limit yourself to the ones above.

HLP in supervision

HLP is not just specific to working with clients who have psychological difficulties. The principles can be applied to any situation that is challenging, including the home environment, work or organisational challenges. I have also used HLP in supervision sessions when appropriate and in the past few years have noticed an increase in the number of supervisees who are seeking a spiritual perspective to their clinical work and supervision. I believe that incorporating a spiritual dimension not only facilitates a supervisee's clinical work but also their own personal spiritual journey and growth. I often introduce the idea of mirrors as part of the learning and teaching process, both with my clients and supervisees. This embraces the concept that we are all each other's mirrors in life including our environments and surroundings; everyone and everything can represent a mirror to us and vice versa. For example, if we feel triggered by something that someone else has said or done, then this may be highlighting an inner wound within oneself. By identifying the wound, there is a chance to heal the theme that wound represents. Once healed and the learning has been integrated, the theme of the wound is no longer triggered. Examples include an instance when a supervisee was feeling stuck with one of their clients, we together explored what the situation was trying to teach, heal, or learn for them and possibly their client. This included identifying areas where the supervisee may be feeling stuck in their life. I have also noticed that it is not uncommon to find a therapist having clusters of clients who present with similar issues, themes, or challenges to what they are currently experiencing in their own life. What is being reflected back to the therapist to help them identify some of their own inner wounds that they can go and explore and heal outside of sessions? Are the messages, support or advice they say to their clients also relevant to themselves and are they practising what they preach and being authentic? As a supervisor, I am also holding in mind the transference and countertransference in my supervision sessions. What are my supervisees mirroring back to me that I need to work on within myself? When you start opening up to this perspective you realise that every relationship in your life is rich with information and guidance for one's own spiritual journey and evolution.

I have also applied HLP when supervisees are struggling with organisational difficulties, in order to facilitate them in understanding what they could learn from such systemic challenges. Teaching supervisees to notice the different messages from their ego, heart, and soul can help them to respect and honour their heart and soul, rather than feel bound by the ego's hooks and expectations. This may enable supervisees to have a healthier outlook on their work circumstances in order to make informed decisions that feel more authentic to them.

The future of HLP

HLP is a new psychotherapy and while based on spiritually informed beliefs, it currently lacks empirical research. It is also immensely difficult to scientifically prove spiritual beliefs! I have presented a few cases throughout this book and elsewhere (Dent, 2025), but obviously moving forward, more research is required. I will continue to collect and record data as I work with my clients, but I am hoping that in the future there will be qualitative and quantitative studies that can show how clients benefit from using HLP as part of a BioPsychoSocioSpiritual approach to treating psychological distress. Qualitative studies comparing the findings from soul therapies, such as the Akashic Records, with independent psychological assessments to identify similarities between past life and current life challenges would also be beneficial.

Summary

- By learning to apply HLP to their lives, clients can hopefully begin to recognise challenges more quickly, make new choices from their heart and soul, rather than their ego, experience less psychological distress, and embrace a more authentic life.
- It is important to make sure your client is stable and not actively psychotic, actively suicidal, highly dissociative or have complex personality difficulties so that they can engage in the concepts and follow the process of HLP.
- During a spiritual journey, clients may experience 'awakening' symptoms including physical and emotional symptoms.
- It is important to look after yourself as a therapist, as well as the environment you work within.
- HLP can be used in supervision to support supervisees with various challenges they may be experiencing including with their clients and organisational issues.

Part 4

Case studies

10

Client and supervisee case studies

Out of suffering have emerged the strongest souls; the most massive characters are seared with scars.

Kahlil Gibran

Three client case studies are now going to be presented to demonstrate how a Bio-PsychoSocioSpiritual model can be used to treat trauma. The first case, Marie, is an example of using HLP informed EMDR. This is illustrated by providing some transcripts of EMDR processing sessions to demonstrate how the Heart Led model of HLP facilitated the processing of traumas, including the use of spiritual interweaves. The second case, Kim, demonstrates how being open to spirituality enabled a client using EMDR to process the recent death of her daughter (transcripts of sessions are provided), in combination with Akashic Record healing, to clear soul level blocks and restrictions. The third case, Alice, is an example of using the HASL model to treat traumas. Alice's initial assessment is detailed along with the work that she undertook with me as well as findings from her Akashic Records. Finally, I discuss part of a supervision session with one of my supervisees and how my openness to spirituality acted as a catalyst for her to reconnect with her own spirituality so that she can start embracing this within her clinical work.

The Akashic Record work reported in the case studies was carried out by my spiritual colleague, Liz King, the process of which was described in more detail in Chapter 8. Liz would have known very little about the clients before seeing them (except their birth name, date of birth, and place of birth), which in many ways is important so that she is not influenced by their stories. Liz would have received permission from the client to access their soul's Akashic Records in the fifth dimension, identify their soul blocks and restrictions and the story behind such difficulties. The clients would then have had a session with Liz to discover what had been found. Liz would then check with the client that the information provided resonated with the client and their current life circumstances. After the session, Liz would then proceed to clear the blocks and restrictions. The information has been voluntarily provided to me by my clients who have reported that it resonated with their own spiritual beliefs and their current lifetime circumstances and that they

DOI: 10.4324/9781003613749-14

have found the clearing work of soul blocks and restrictions highly beneficial. It is important to highlight that there is no scientific proof or evidence to support or verify any of the Akashic Record information reported in the case studies and it is based on spiritual beliefs rather than facts.

Case study 1: Marie

First Marie's background history will be presented followed by two transcripts of EMDR sessions, which will highlight how her awareness of HLP facilitated her into moving from her ego into her heart during EMDR processing. Her transcripts also provide indications of her possible primary life lesson.

Marie was a lady in her mid-50s who had been an inpatient on a psychiatric ward the year before our initial appointment, where she was diagnosed with Emotionally Unstable Personality Disorder and depression. Her follow-up support from the National Health Service (NHS) was minimal and she was heavily medicated on Aripiprazole (anti-psychotic), Escitalopram (anti-depressant), Clonazepam (for her benign tremor), and Zopiclone (sleeping tablet). When I first met her she was actively suicidal, but keen to regain control of her life and start 'feeling' again, reporting that she had been numb to all emotions since her psychiatric admission.

Her recollection of her childhood was minimal. She had two brothers who were favoured and while she acknowledged that her physical needs were met, there was no love or nurturance from her parents. She described her mother as 'nutty as a fruit cake' with low mood and anger issues. She said her mother found it hard to parent a daughter and didn't trust Marie. This resulted in Marie having subsequent trust issues and never feeling accepted for who she was, which ultimately made it hard for her to accept herself. Her father had anger issues and would 'thrash' the children. Marie recognised that she was emotionally shut down as a child and that she still struggled to accept positive emotions from anyone. She attempted suicide during her teens. Marie's attendance at school was minimal. Positive nurturing figures in her life included her maternal grandad and great-grandmother.

Marie met her husband when she was 15 years old and he came from a loving and supportive family. Marie went to college and left home when 16 years old, then found a job and bought her own flat, which is where she lived for three years before getting married. This was a very positive time for her. Once married, Marie fell pregnant with her first child. She worked part-time after having her daughter and her son was born four years later. A few years later she discovered her husband had a brief affair with a close friend, which devastated her. She stayed with her husband and children but did report struggling with her emotions and feeling very low at times.

In 2016, Marie's father became terminally ill with cancer and she decided that she would care for him until he died. Also, during this time, her son was diagnosed with Bipolar Disorder and attempted suicide twice and she has since lived in fear of one day losing him. Toward the end of 2016, Marie said that her difficulties became very apparent. She didn't realise at the time the impact that her father's death was having on her and she struggled to grieve for him. She spent most of 2017 in and out of psychiatric hospital, as she was very emotionally unstable and suicidal. Marie had decided to live independently from her husband and their son due to her own and her son's psychological issues.

Marie came with a significant trauma and attachment history and no one had ever helped her to understand her difficulties from this perspective, so when I formulated it in this way she kept saying 'That makes so much sense.' Marie's score on the Impact Event Scale – Revised (IES-R; Weiss & Marmar, 1996) was 58, which is above the suggested cut-off score of 33 for a probable diagnosis of PTSD. Marie completed the Patient Health Questionnaire – Somatic, Anxiety, and Depressive Symptoms (PHQ-SADS; Kroneke, Spitzer, Williams, & Lowe, 2010). Her score on the PHQ-15 sub-section was 11, which is suggestive of medium somatic symptom severity; her score on the Patient Health Questionnaire-9 (PHQ-9) was 25, suggestive of severe depressive symptoms; and she scored 15 on the sub-section Generalised Anxiety Disorder Assessment (GAD-7) suggesting severe anxiety symptoms (Spitzer, Kroenke, Williams, & Lowe, 2006). On the PTSD Checklist (PCL-5; Blevins, Weathers, Davis, Witte, & Domino, 2015), Marie scored 45 (cut-off of 33) indicating further assessment for a diagnosis of PTSD.

After our first appointment, Marie decided with her psychiatrist to come off her anti-psychotic medication as she wasn't finding it was adding any benefit. Having completed a risk assessment, we then went through some psychoeducation as well as mindfulness, mindful breathing, resource strategies, positive affirmations, and also worked on improving her diet and daily activities. We then went through the HL model. Before commencing EMDR processing, we had one session using Ego State work to meet and engage her 'protective part.' Marie found this a very positive session and reported feeling much stronger in herself afterwards. She was also utilising all of the resource strategies she had been taught and said others were reporting noticing the positive changes in her too.

While Marie had many traumas in her past, the area she really wanted to focus on first was her husband's affair, as she felt this was having the most effect on her currently and was impacting on her ability to trust him. I have transcribed two of our sessions to demonstrate how the concepts of the HL model can facilitate processing. The worst moment was the image of her husband telling her about the affair. Her negative cognition was 'I am not good enough' with the preferred belief being 'I am a good person' with VOC 2/7. She felt upset and angry, her SUDS were 8/10 and she felt this in her stomach. After each BLS, I asked Marie 'What did you notice?' and her feedback is detailed below. After her response, I simply said 'Go with that.'

- Stomach is a bit better. It was so long ago. I shouldn't let it affect me like this.
- I want to trust him. I can trust him. I've got to trust him.
- Why did he hurt me? I can trust him now, he is such a lovely person.
- Angry with myself because I feel guilty about not trusting him. I've still got that doubt there.
- Let me believe in myself and not feel guilty. It upsets me that I feel guilty.
- I need to let the guilt go and be my old self.
- He's such a lovely person. I've got to start standing up for myself and not feel guilty if I say no to him.
- This is the second time I've lost his trust but does it really matter now? Take him as he is now, he is the man I married.
- I've got to be stronger in myself, and be honest with him if I don't want to do something. I need to believe in myself.
- I'm trying to be rational. I shouldn't feel guilty. He says he loves me, I need to accept this. If I start saying no to him sometimes and he doesn't like it, then I'll know he's not for me.
- I've lost some best friends because of him. I need to let it go. He is my best friend.
- I love him and don't want to lose him but I've got to live my life and be me, but I am not sure who me is.

At this stage I felt Marie's ego was in control, so I just asked Marie to bring her awareness into her heart, notice what her heart was trying to communicate to her and then I restarted BLS.

- I am not losing him. My head is saying I must love him but I don't know how to do that. I can erase the affair out of my head but my heart is saying I don't trust him.

During this set Marie started to cry for the first time in several years, so I continued the BLS for a longer time to enable her to really process her sadness.

- I must love him in my heart.
- My head is ruling my heart. I need to start going more into my heart.
- My heart is beating fast. I do over-analyse things. I need to think more with my heart.

This session was incomplete, so before we finished I asked her what the most important thing she had learned from the processing. Marie said, 'I can choose to live life through my heart.' I installed this using some BLS and this belief became stronger. When Marie moved into her heart she was able to connect with her sadness for the first time in many years. This was very significant for her and helped her to believe she could express emotions.

When I met Marie a week later, she told me that she had a very positive week. Despite taking several days to build up the confidence, she managed to speak to her husband and have a heart-to-heart about her fears. She felt this was a huge step forward, but also she was starting to feel happy for the first time in many years. Her SUDS from the session before were down to 3/10 so we continued processing the memory. The image of the worst moment had changed slightly to that of imagining her children upstairs while the affair was happening downstairs. Her negative cognition was 'I am a failure' with the preferred cognition being 'I am a good person' with VOC 2/7. She felt tearful and angry in her stomach.

- I am telling myself we have been together all these years so I can't be a failure.
- I am almost laughing inside, none of us are perfect and maybe it was a heat of the moment for him.
- It has been ruining my life and I need to get rid of it. He said it won't happen again.
- The last few months he has proven that he loves me. My ego is saying I fear losing him. My heart is saying I am not going to lose him.
- I've got to be stronger with my heart than my head as he is a loving, kind person and would do anything for anyone. There is still a wedge between us regarding our son, but I need to accept this with my heart and not let it ruin what we have.
- Thinking more about the wedge between us regarding my son and I have got to accept that it is how things are. I want to help him (son) but he won't let anyone help him. Fear that I could lose him (son) at any moment. But he (son) doesn't let either of us in so I have to accept this is the way he is and not let it drive a wedge between us.
- It's only me distressing myself over it. I've got to deal with it. I feel guilty – I have got to get rid of this.
- I will accept myself and talk about it rather than ignore it, as my heart wants to say things.

At this point Marie had a few tears in her eyes.

- If I carry on like this and speak from my heart I can do this compared to having mixed-up feelings in my head.

- I can accept myself. I am not second best to my husband. I felt he chose my son over me. I now understand his reasons because he is his dad.
- Thinking back to when it all happened. I wasn't in a good place. I thought I was coping but in hindsight I was putting a protective shield up as I was so wrapped up with my dad. Guilty. But my husband and son kept me out of the equation (when the son attempted suicide) and my husband has apologised since. What we are doing now is for our son. I have to accept that life doesn't pan out the way you expect. I need to go with how it is. It is a good thing to let go of the guilt. It has been better over the past few months.
- I held back on having a conversation with my son in the past because it led to arguments. What I need to do is talk to him. I need to ask him how his day has been instead of feeling guilty. I can accept the situation as it is. I am doing this for my son. I am not second best, I need to accept this, and then things can progress forward.
- When I think through my heart, it comes out right. When I think through my head it goes wrong. It's up to them (husband and son) if they like me for who I am.
- I don't think black and white now or over-analyse. Therefore I should use my heart and not my head so that I don't over-analyse and get things wrong.

This session was incomplete, so before we finished I asked her what the most important thing she had learned from the processing. Marie said, 'I am a good person.' I installed this using some BLS and this belief became stronger. What was really interesting in this session was that Marie was applying the ideas of HLP on her own and recognising how she would progress if she started trusting her heart and not her ego. There was also a noticeable theme about ACCEPTANCE that kept coming through in her responses during BLS sets. At the end of the session, we reflected on whether this could be part of her life lesson and related this to her experiences throughout her life, where she didn't feel accepted by her parents and then didn't accept herself at many times, including difficulty accepting positive emotions from her husband and children. In the transcript above she mentioned wanting to accept herself and accept the situation between her and her son, as well as accepting her husband's affair, accept that she can let go of her guilt so that she could free herself up from the distress and become more authentic in herself. At the following session, Marie reported that the memory was no longer distressing, SUDS 0/10 so we installed her positive cognition, which had changed to 'I am strong enough' and had a VOC of 7/7 (completely true). Her body scan was clear.

   I continued to work with Marie to help her process the trauma of her earlier relationship with her father, the death of her father, her son's attempted suicides and her attempted suicides. We had 12 sessions in total over four months, five of which were EMDR sessions processing past traumas. All of these memories were processed to completion. At the end of therapy, Marie's score on the IES-R was 18 (down from 58). On the PHQ-SADS, her score on the PHQ-15 sub-section was 3 (previously 11); PHQ-9 was 1 (previously 25) and GAD-7 score was 3 (previously 15). On the PCL-5 Marie scored 6 (previously 45). All of her scores were within normal range and showed a drastic overall improvement.

Marie continued to have the theme of acceptance running through her feedback during the desensitisation phase and when she connected with her heart she was able to process her emotions and also start accepting love from her son, believing that she was a good mother for the first time in her life. Not only was Marie learning to embrace living life through her heart, she was also relieved that she was starting to experience emotions again which had such a positive impact on her and her acceptance of herself. She was keen to wean herself off her anti-depressant medication too.

Case study 2: Kim

This case demonstrates the benefits of using a BioPsychoSocioSpiritual approach when working with traumas to facilitate multi-dimensional healing. First, I will give you a background to the case from this current lifetime, before illustrating some transcribed EMDR sessions with Kim, to show how EMDR processing can facilitate healing at a very spiritual level. Finally I will summarise Kim's soul level blocks and restrictions based on information provided during her Akashic Record work.

Kim's current lifetime

Kim was a lady in her mid-40s who had been seeing another psychologist for three years due to long-standing anxiety and while she had made some progress she was still struggling on most days. Kim had mentioned to her psychologist that her son, Fred, was also struggling with anxiety, in particular OCD symptoms, and my services were recommended to help with her son.

Kim initially contacted me several months before committing to an appointment. The deciding factor was the tragic and sudden death of her 19-year-old daughter, Sarah, a month earlier. Kim brought her son, Fred, to an appointment and told me how Sarah had suffered from diabetes since she was one year old and how this had triggered Kim's anxiety. Fred had always been the 'perfect child,' unlike Sarah, who had been much more challenging, especially during her teenage years. Fred and Sarah were half-siblings but had been very close.

I saw Fred for a few sessions to support him with his anxiety. What was apparent is that he reported feeling more relaxed when he was on his own, rather than when his parents were around. Fred started to make some progress and found using distractions beneficial when managing his anxiety. However, I remained concerned about home life and his anxiety in relation to his parents, especially his mother. I arranged an appointment with just his parents so that we could discuss the dynamics and how we could support Kim with her own anxiety. My feeling was that if Kim's anxiety improved, so would Fred's.

When I met Kim and her husband they were very receptive to trying to resolve their own issues and could recognise the impact these were having on Fred. Kim told me that she had always worried about her children's health ever since they were born and expressed concerns that she had 'created Fred's issues.' She told me that she had regularly checked Fred's neck for any signs of lumps on a daily basis throughout his life. Since the death of Sarah, Fred had been Kim's main comfort. She disclosed how her anxieties dated back to her childhood where she had never been contained by her own mother.

Independently and based on my recommendation, Kim had been to see my spiritualist colleague, Liz King for a psychic reading. I therefore discussed with Kim the possibility of her undertaking some Akashic Record work to clear any potential soul level blocks and restrictions between her and Fred, because I intuitively sensed that something was making it very difficult for her to parent him. Kim went ahead with completing her own Akashic Records, Fred's, Sarah's, and her husband's, and an overlay between each different member of the family.

At the same time Kim expressed interest in having some sessions with myself to try and get to the root cause of her anxiety. From my assessment of Kim, it was apparent that there were lots of unprocessed memories from when Kim had felt abandoned and rejected by her parents growing up, so I explained how EMDR could help process her early memories. After teaching Kim some resources and mindfulness, we used EMDR to process a memory of when she was three years old. At the following session, Kim asked to process Sarah's death (which by this time had occurred six months earlier). I have transcribed three of our EMDR sessions to highlight how being open to spirituality can really benefit processing.

We identified the worst moment of the memory in relation to Sarah's death. The image was of Sarah in the morgue and the negative cognition was 'I have failed.' The preferred cognition was 'I did the best I could' with a VOC of 1/7 and the resulting emotions were sadness and anger. The subjective unit of distress was 10/10 which she felt in her head.

The following are responses Kim gave after each set of BLS. As you will observe, during the processing Kim is communicating with Sarah's spirit in imagination. Sarah's spirit was acting as a facilitator to Kim to help Kim make sense of what happened and come to terms with Sarah's death. I didn't need to use any interweaves (Sarah's spirit is managing to do this when required!) so between each set I would just say 'notice that.'

- Feeling upset. I am angry with the detectives. Parts of her body are hard to look at. I dragged her body into the car (in imagination).
- I got in the car, shouted at Fred to get in, and then out again. I am driving away with Sarah's body in the back seat. Her spirit is sitting next to me in the passenger seat, laughing, saying 'I am not here. Take me back.'
- I pulled the car over and shouted a lot. I dragged her body out of the car and tried cardiopulmonary resuscitation. She is watching me, telling me she doesn't want to go back to how she was. She tells me she is still with me in spirit but not physically and I need to accept this.
- We had a big row. I asked her why she chose this path. She said she didn't have an option. She is saying she is happier now but unhappy because I am unhappy. She shouts, 'Sort your shit out!'
- We get to a resolution of the argument. She said, 'I've been brought out of this life to go to the next one. If you open your mind, you will be enlightened and we can enjoy the next lifetime together. I won't have to be ill next time.'
- We get back into the car and I drive back to the morgue. I asked her, 'How do I get to see you?' She said, 'I am always here, always around and part of you. Fred is the key and we all have to support him. His purity has to spread.' I still don't get an apology from her for dying!
- We are arguing again in the car, I am accusing her of doing this to us. She is saying she is not sorry, it isn't real, it doesn't matter. It doesn't exist. The only thing is life. She said, 'What is your problem?' I told her she should apologise for dying and that she had made me fearful of death.
- I pulled over again. I said, 'I understand but it's all really hard.' She put her hand on my arm and said 'You are not without me, I am still here, I am not going anywhere. We have to take the body back.'
- She is in the back of the car, hitting her body saying, 'See, it's not real. I wasn't there the day before I died, my spirit had left my body. I wanted to call you but didn't.'
- Sarah said, 'It wasn't me, I wasn't there. It's just crap. But get rid of this piece of shit' (dancing on top of her body).
- There is a song she is singing. I pulled into the morgue and they take the body away. She said, 'The point is, I need you to do this for me. You've

got to get with the programme, there is a bigger thing going on here.' She linked arms with Fred and my husband and said 'We are a family.'

The session finished incomplete, so before we concluded I asked what was the most important thing she had learned from the processing. Kim said, 'I believe I have the strength to do what needs to be done.' I installed this using some BLS and her belief changed to 'I can do it. I will do it.'

At the next session we reviewed the processing from the week before and the SUDS had come down to 2/10 and Kim didn't feel the distress would decrease below this, because of the reality of having lost her daughter. In certain situations, especially where there is complicated grief, it is accepted that the SUDS levels may never reach 0/10 and therefore a slightly higher SUD score is accepted (known as ecological validity). Kim was also keen to move on and process the time when she had heard about Sarah's death. The target image was her husband walking through the office door. Her negative cognition was 'I have failed' and the positive cognition was 'I can learn to get through this' with a VOC of 2/7. She felt terror, her SUDS were 10/10, which was felt in her head. As with before, Sarah's spirit came into the processing in imagination. I kept out of the way and just asked her to 'notice that' in between BLS sets.

- Seeing Sarah leaning over the morgue crying and saying, 'What have I done?'
- She then burst out of the morgue roof crying, 'I need to get to my mummy.' She came into our bedroom that night, floated around, and then turned into the dog and started licking our faces and being very attentive.
- I picked up my sister the next day and Sarah's spirit comes with us in the car to the morgue, angry. We get to the morgue. Sarah is seeing the white light but says, 'I am not ready.' She screams at me to get out of the morgue, which I do and she is resisting the white light.
- She is flitting between different people, friends, etc. Also sitting with her head in her hands.
- She decides to walk home, crawl into bed with us, cuddling. The white light is there and coming closer. She is resisting although knows it is going to happen.
- Her spiritual guide has come to explain what is happening. She is told that my husband is her soul father and this is all part of his lesson too. She is still resisting. She is told she needed to die for Fred to do good things.
- Her spirit guide is telling her that she is needed back as she is a nanny to younger souls, she was never meant to live this long. He starts touching and healing her. He tells her she can come back at any stage (spiritually).

- She got halfway through the white light then ran back and kissed us. She is now being reunited with her soul group but still struggling to get her head around it all.

This session again was incomplete, so before we finished I asked what was the most important thing she had learned from the processing. Kim said, 'I can learn to see or accept the bigger picture.' As I installed this using some BLS her belief changed to 'I can learn to believe.' The next session we continued processing this memory to completion, which involved Kim having a conversation with Sarah's spirit about what to do with her ashes.

The following EMDR session was spent processing the worst time that Kim was anxious as a child. The image was of her mother cowering in the room and Kim's dad standing over her. Her negative cognition was 'I am not safe' with the preferred cognition being 'I am safe now' with VOC 2/7. She felt anxious and angry, her SUDS were 7/10 which were felt in her stomach. Although Sarah hadn't been born at this stage, her spirit came into the process guiding Kim within this childhood memory.

- I am frozen. Sarah is sitting on the bed cross-legged saying, 'Let's look at this.'
- Sarah started discussing times when I had fought with my husband and how I had also been scared as a child when in this situation of observing my parents fighting.

Kim then connected to her childhood memory.

- I am scared that my dad will hurt me more than mum. I didn't get a chance to leave whereas mum managed to sever all ties. Sarah is saying that my dad is spiritually wanting to talk to me.
- I was bullied all childhood, I had no control. I had to ask for everything including food. I was not allowed to be in control. My dad was a bully. I always tried to make him happy. I have done the same to Fred with my anxiety and controlling his childhood.
- Sarah said, 'It's not your fault, it is who he is (Fred), he just wants you to be happy. Once that is achieved he will be free of this. I chose my death as quick as possible as I didn't want a long painful death. You need to trust and accept that it is all for your highest good. Let go and Fred will follow.'
- Sarah continued talking to me saying, 'Trust. There is nothing you can do that will change it. You have to experience it and not control where it ends. Accept each day as it comes. Your dad is still wanting to speak to you!'
- I opened the door to allow my dad to come in and he started crying. He was hugging Sarah. He said sorry to me. His life lesson was about loss. He lost everything.

- He is telling me he realised he didn't behave well. He has had to do things spiritually since to realise this.
- He is telling me to learn to let it go. Sarah was sent to cause stress, grief and love but ultimately to know that it is OK. My mother is the same. Dad tells me he has karma with my mum.

Again, the session was incomplete, but we finished by installing what Kim had learned from the session processing, which was 'I can learn to trust and accept.' As we processed this, the belief got stronger and included learning to love.

Kim and I continued working together to process her distressing memories using EMDR. I had no idea before starting to process what was going to happen, so I just held the space for her to start healing spiritually. Kim believed it was Sarah's spirit speaking to her because she said Sarah was as feisty in spirit as she had been when alive. Sarah's spirit was also guiding Kim using imaginary scenarios with areas that were particularly difficult for Kim to come to terms with, in particular, the acceptance of Sarah's death and Fred's spiritual role in Kim's life. When I have used EMDR with complicated grief, other clients have noticed how a light stream enters the room at pertinent points which has given them a sense of comfort.

Kim's Akashic Records

The information below was provided to me by Kim based on what she was told during her Akashic Record healing with my spiritual colleague, although there is no way of verifying the validity of what she was told. However, Kim reported that this information resonated with her.

1   Kim's Akashic Records

Kim's life lesson is about inner authority. Kim had a soulmate contract with Sarah to repair her. There was a strong possibility that Sarah had previously been Kim's son in a past life, but that her son had been taken away from her. This had created negative unjustified karma. Kim had made two vows, one of sacrifice and one of suffering to save her children. She had a witch's wound and experienced soul facet loss. She had a perception that everyone was always right and not her. She also had a constant anticipation about loss, due to her past life experiences.

2   Sarah's Akashic Records

Kim was told that Sarah's life lesson was happiness. Sarah's soul is a natural healer and teacher and is known as a nanny of the souls and she has a very high spiritual vibration. She was one of three sisters selected to protect a chosen child in Egypt, but the child was lost and Sarah always blamed herself for this, carrying unjustified negative karma, which is about penitence. Sarah had made three vows in the past; sacrifice, suffering, and silence. Sarah had been bound to restrict her healing abilities and had experienced some soul facet loss. Kim was told that Sarah also had four tares on her chakras; sacral, heart, throat, and third eye chakras.

3   Joint overlay between Kim and Sarah Akashic Records

Kim and Sarah are twin souls and have a joint lesson of courage. There is a vow of sacrifice between them and a karmic imprint sitting at the heart chakra from eight lifetimes ago. Sarah's binding had taken away her soul and Divine power and she is still trying to save Fred. Sarah was called back from her physical body to be a guide and teacher to younger souls. Her death was pre-determined, she was never meant to live older than her 20s.

Summary of Kim

Kim reported that she really benefitted from the EMDR sessions and that although there was recognition that life would always be tough, the EMDR helped her feel stronger and start understanding the bigger picture rather than getting caught up with the ego, which was making her feel the victim. Her anxiety lessened especially in relation to Fred. She reported that the Akashic Records work not only gave her some insight into her soul level blocks and restrictions, but clearing these helped Kim, as well as her relationships with family members, so that she could make new conscious choices at a heart and soul level. It also helped her to possibly understand why she had always had a fear of losing her children. A year later when I contacted Kim she reported that the benefits of both the psychological intervention and her Akashic Record clearing were still holding. Fred was doing well at school and was much less anxious in general.

Case study 3: Alice

In this third case study, I will describe Alice's initial assessment in detail and how I used HLP informed EMDR (using the HASL model) to heal her traumas, which also helped identify her probable primary life lesson. I will then summarise Alice's blocks and restrictions identified from her Akashic Records demonstrating how Alice was healing multi-dimensionally.
Alice's current life

The initial assessment was completed over three sessions. It required this length of time because during the first session Alice recounted a detailed narrative of the past three traumatic years of her life, which involved the birth of her two children and their serious physical health issues. The subsequent two sessions focused on her background history as well as exploring spirituality and the HASL model.

Alice discussed how her three-year-old son, Charlie, had many health issues during his first year of life and had been hospitalised eight times. On his first birthday, Charlie was diagnosed with Kawasaki Heart Disease and had inflamed pulmonary arteries. He was left with a weakened immune system and needed regular appointments with a cardiologist. Charlie was subsequently admitted with pneumonia and at one point tested for leukaemia. At this time, Alice was five months pregnant with her second child. Alice was closely monitored during her second pregnancy, but all investigations were found to be clear. Alice had her second child, Sophie, at home naturally. The midwife detected an initial heart murmur but didn't have any more concerns. That night, Alice became anxious about Sophie's breathing and when she checked, noticed her daughter's feet were dark purple. Alice called for an ambulance and Sophie was taken to hospital where she needed to be resuscitated and was diagnosed with sepsis. Sophie was kept in hospital that night and during this time the cardiologist responsible for Charlie heard about Sophie's situation and completed an assessment immediately. Sophie was diagnosed with a rare complex heart defect and heart failure (Truncus Arteriosus), which is usually detected prenatally. Sophie was rushed to intensive care at Great Ormond Street Hospital (GOSH) where she was placed on the list for open-heart surgery once a donor heart became available. Alice and her husband stayed in London, leaving Charlie in the care of Alice's mother. After four days of waiting at GOSH, Alice woke up in the early hours with a sudden panic and told her husband that she needed to see Charlie, she couldn't explain why, she just had a mother's intuition that she needed to get back to him. Alice got in the car and drove two hours home only to find Charlie unconscious in his bed. He was rushed to hospital and Alice was told that if she had found Charlie 10 minutes later he would probably have died because his blood sugars were so low. That same day, a donor heart was found for Sophie, who immediately underwent heart surgery. Despite the local hospital's best efforts, they were unable to transfer Charlie to GOSH, so Alice had to make the difficult decision of leaving him in the care of her mother and returning to London.

The outcome of Sophie's surgery was not known for many days – she was critically ill and fighting for her life. Alice described the scene of visiting Sophie for the first time after the operation, completely covered in tubes and machines beeping in the background with multiple professionals frantically rushing around by her bedside. Alice collapsed on the floor and cried out 'Put her back in my tummy.' A compassionate nurse came and explained everything; what all the equipment was for and what support Sophie was being given, which helped Alice feel more trusting of the professionals.

Alice had not only given birth four days earlier but she had no time to recover before experiencing trauma after trauma, nearly losing both her children. She was exhausted, trying to express milk for her daughter, and was in survival mode. She was not allowed to hold Sophie for the first 42 days. A kind friend set up a Just Giving account to raise money so that Alice and her family could afford to rent a flat opposite GOSH and they remained in London for three months – Charlie was able to join when he was better, and Alice and her husband were determined to try and keep everything as normal as possible for Charlie, while also caring for Sophie.

I heard how Sophie is going to need at least three further heart operations in the near future. Alice's score on the IES-R was 81 (maximum score obtainable is 88), which suggested she was still very traumatised from the past three years. She scored 8 on the PHQ-9 (Kroenke, Spitzer, & Williams, 2001), which is below the cut-off required for suggesting depressive symptoms and 14 on the GAD-7 suggesting moderate anxiety symptoms (Spitzer et al., 2006). The Mindfulness Attention Awareness Scale (MAAS) (Brown & Ryan, 2003) is a 15-item questionnaire that assesses dispositional mindfulness, in other words an individual's awareness of being in the present moment. The minimum score possible is 15 with a maximum score of 90. The higher the score, the more mindful the individual. Alice's score was 45 suggesting that she is somewhat mindful in life.

I was struck by how emotional I felt listening to Alice's narrative (at times fighting back the tears), while she was able to sit opposite me rather calmly and matter-of-factly and discuss the details of what she had been through. I was acutely aware of myself and how I was picking up the transference of Alice's emotions. I was also struck during this session by how my body felt, I had tingling in my head, neck, and shoulders at certain points during her narrative, a bit like shivers through parts of my body. These were at very significant points, including when she described how she had a 'knowing' of checking on her children at different intervals, having saved both their lives. I believe that these were signs for me to recognise possible spiritual opportunities and such phenomena have also been reported by other therapists during sessions (e.g. Siegel, 2018). Most therapists may not experience a physical reaction, but I have noticed that as my spiritual resonance with clients is strengthening in momentum, so is my awareness of signs, which sometimes come via physical sensations or intuitive thoughts during sessions.

Discussing Alice's background history, I learned how Alice's father had been physically abusive to her between the ages of two and 15 years old, with the intensity increasing from eight years old. She witnessed him being abusive to her mother, including him attempting to run her mother over in the car. Alice was raped when she was 15 years old and self-harmed around this time, ending up in hospital with a fractured jawbone from her father. She was put on the child-at-risk register, but the physical abuse continued and her mother just kept her at home when she had been beaten in order to hide the abuse from school. Alice also attempted suicide around this time. Her mother finally filed for a divorce but this was very stressful and involved a lot of lying and coercion from her father with the authorities and her mother tried to commit suicide with the strain of it all. Despite having some intervention from CAMHS, she didn't get much relief from therapy. Alice left home when she was 16 years old, moved away to complete a fashion course and this is when she met her husband and they married nine years later. When Alice left her family home she cut all communication with her father for three years, but later decided to lower expectations of him and very slowly managed to rebuild a relationship to the extent that she asked him to give her away at her wedding. Soon after marrying, Alice miscarried, was diagnosed with polycystic ovarian syndrome and was told it would be difficult for her to conceive. Fortunately, four years after this Charlie was born and Sophie arrived 18 months later. On both Alice and her husband's side of the family there were psychological difficulties as well as complex relationships between family members.

Not surprisingly, Alice commented to me that she was finding everyday interactions with people difficult, listening to their general complaints and worries about life when she has experienced so much distress and trauma. She believed that she was on borrowed time with Sophie but tried to turn this into a positive by cherishing each moment. In spite of all of this, she had set up and been running her own successful business with her husband for 10 years and between the two of them, they took responsibility for their children's childcare. Due to the children's health issues, the family was restricted to what they could do as they could not afford for their children to become unwell. While Alice had a close relationship with her mother, there were infrequent face-to-face interactions, as her mother had been suffering from lymphoma for seven years and had decided not to have any further treatment. This meant that her mother had a weakened immune system and was susceptible to viruses.

During the assessment phase there was an opportunity to look at spirituality when Alice mentioned that she was keen to start doing some yoga and meditation again. At this point I simply asked what her spiritual beliefs were. It was like watching Pandora's Box open, she quickly told me how interested she was in spirituality, including at a soul level. We began to discuss the HASL model and formulate how it could relate to her life and challenges and agreed an initial treatment plan with the option of possible soul therapy with my spiritual colleague. During this conversation, the energy in the room was immense. Alice told me she had recently written a letter on a website called Hi Mama (Alice gave me permission to include this below). Exploring spirituality not only gave Alice a sense of hope but also linked in with the spiritual perspective she was taking on life about identifying the gifts within every challenge.

In formulating Alice's situation using a HASL model, it is evident that she had early blocks and restrictions from the abuse of her father. With complex family relationships, these could be indicators of soul blocks and restrictions. While she had a close relationship with her mother, her mother was unable to protect her or keep her safe growing up. Alice's trust in individuals growing up was minimal. She had to shut down her emotional part of herself when she was little because life was frightening and unpredictable. No significant dissociative symptoms were evident on the Dissociative Experience Scale (DES) (Bernstein & Putnam, 1986). Alice's ongoing challenges were evident, but what was more apparent was her strength and determination. It is not uncommon for a strong person to experience complex traumas and challenges so that they can learn their life lessons – otherwise, it would be too easy for them! Making new choices and taking leaps of faith is very hard to do. Sometimes, the stronger and more able the soul, the tougher the challenges and traumas.

Alice was already very spiritually minded when we met. However, ongoing life challenges meant this part of her life was 'parked' to one side. As you will see below from the letter she wrote, Alice had great insight and awareness and could recognise gifts from her traumas. Part of my role in working with Alice was to re-ignite her spirituality. In addition to learning to live her life through her heart and soul, we built up her resources and coping strategies, teaching her to be more mindful and learning how to engage with her emotions so that her window of tolerance increased. We then processed her recent traumas using EMDR, particularly the birth of Sophie and hospitalisations with Charlie, as this was causing Alice the most distress in her life. While Alice had some very insightful knowledge, she sometimes struggled to put this into practice with everyday challenges. Therefore, as required, a few sessions focused specifically on HLP, helping her re-evaluate her work commitments against family responsibilities and her own well-being. During the EMDR processing, Alice identified that the primary life lesson that resonated with her was SURRENDER, letting go of needing to control everything and start becoming calmer in herself. Holding on to this idea of surrender really helped her make new choices as it gave her a different approach to managing the ongoing uncertain health issues with her children. Alice's questionnaire scores three months after starting therapy showed a dramatic improvement. Having used HLP informed EMDR to process her daughter's birth, her score on the IES-R was 21, which is significantly lower than before (previously 81). She scored 4 on the PHQ-9 (previously 8) and 7 on the GAD-7 (previously 14). Her score on the MAAS had increased from 45 to 72, suggesting that she was much more mindful than when previously assessed a few months earlier (maximum score possible is 90).

Alice once told me:

> We were definitely supposed to meet, without doubt. If I hadn't been through this situation, if you didn't offer EMDR our paths may not have crossed. I love the path of life and how souls cross to give messages and insights to each other.

Here is Alice's letter that she wrote about her experiences of having Sophie.

Letter to the mama of a broken-hearted baby

Hi mama,

You've just been told your baby has a broken heart. Your whole world has fallen to pieces and you feel like your own heart is in smithereens, you feel physical pain in your own chest and a sinking, dreaded feeling like never before. Right now you feel as though your world has ended, you will spend every waking minute from here on worrying about the 'what ifs' and you will come so close to giving up, but know this: whatever life throws at you, you WILL get through this, life will just be very different from here on.

You should be at home, in that newborn euphoria, cuddling her, feeding her, getting to know her, recovering ... but instead here you are in intensive care, sat crying as you watch her motionless, desperate to see her eyes open, to grasp your finger, to hold her, to change her nappy, to wash her clothes. Your time will come and when it does every normal thing will feel like a miraculous event. It will be magical.

Right now your mind is filled with a thousand questions, you can't sleep a wink for thinking of all possible outcomes. From here on your mind will never rest, you will never stop questioning, wondering, hoping and praying. Her future is very uncertain, you hate that. You are told her condition is life-limiting and you are crushed to your core. You are told there is a chance she won't make it through her surgery and if she does she will be lucky to make it through her childhood and if she does ... it's a life filled with multiple open-heart surgeries, catheter procedures, endless blood tests, heart scans, hospital appointments, medications, and restrictions. It's not the life you imagined for her, for you, for her brother, for the rest of the family and you will grieve a lot. But soon, this will become your 'new normal' and you will take comfort from knowing that she won't know any different and neither will your son. You will make the right decisions for them, for you all.

Soon the days of pre-congenital heart disease will become hazy. You'll not have much time to think about or miss those days yet at the same time you will never want to go back to a time without her; you cannot imagine not seeing her smile, so don't wish your time away, instead learn to cherish her, to cherish time, to cherish every single minuscule moment as a family of four and as crazy as this sounds, you'll start to realise you're lucky. You are fortunate. You are not to be pitied, but envied as you have been given a gift. A gift which has given you a totally different perspective on life; a different perspective on having children. You will learn to appreciate every, single, little thing; the things other mothers take for granted; the natural rise and fall of your children's chests, the beating of their hearts, the warmth of their skin, the weight of their bodies in your arms. You'll be so very grateful for all these seemingly normal things because these are the things you once thought you'd never see or feel again.

I know right now you feel like a mere shadow of your former self. Your light that once lit up a room has gone out but don't worry because that light isn't gone, it's just been passed from you to her and when she gets a bit better you'll start to see it. She needs your light and you need her to have it because she will brighten your every day, she will dazzle everyone she meets, she will light up the darkness that engulfs you ... and my goodness how she will shine!

You will live in constant fear of what's to come ... but you will learn to smile through it. You will find a way to laugh through the tears, to embrace the craziness of your newfound life and most of all you will learn to love more than you ever thought possible; each other ... your bubble and the people that surround you.

You're strong-willed and stubborn (she is her mother's daughter for sure!) and I know you don't like to take advice but hear me out ... please! SLOW DOWN! You have your own heart and health to look after too. Your own health will suffer as you sacrifice your all but remember your children and your husband need you ... so looking after them means looking after you too, it's not selfish, it's sensible.

Take time for each other. Your husband has always been your rock but he is about to become your mountain! You'll both find this journey so incredibly hard but you will be so grateful that you're in this together. Don't be afraid to talk to each other for fear of upsetting each other, don't be afraid to cry and admit that you're struggling. Take the time to remind each other how much you mean to each other, aside from being heart parents, you're a couple, a husband and wife. You are also individuals ... make time for each other and give each other time out, it's needed.

Be present. Cry. But never forget to smile and LOVE. Love like there is no tomorrow. Live the best version of your life that you can and have no regrets. Don't wait for second chances, don't put things off, for you will never know what tomorrow will bring. Appreciate each moment, each milestone, and celebrate victories no matter how big or small. And last but not least no matter how busy you are, no matter how tired you feel, no matter how much you fear waking her up always, ALWAYS kiss her goodnight ... be grateful for today and be hopeful for tomorrow. Xx

Alice's Akashic Records

The information below was provided to me by Alice based on what she was told during her Akashic Record healing with my spiritual colleague, Liz King. Although there is no way of verifying the validity of what she was told, Alice reported that this information resonated with her.

1   Current life blocks and restrictions

Liz felt that there was a lot of judgement in Alice's records that was continuing to affect her. During this current lifetime, Alice was told that she had been in receipt of negative thought forms from a father-type figure between the ages of 15 and 18 years old. This would have been at a time when Alice would have been thinking about her independence. Negative thoughts are sent from someone else over a period of time with intention and when they have been sent long enough they can become internalised by the recipient. The negative thought forms were all about passivity, the sender wanting to keep Alice in a box or cage, not allowing her freedom. From 15 years old, Alice would have questioned her independence, and ability to find her voice and feel empowered, especially when in contact with individuals with masculine energy. In addition, negative thought forms were sent more recently, by another person with masculine energy, who had no warmth or caring. This person would have been very challenging, questioning Alice's authority in a very vocal manner (Alice was able to recognise who this person was in her life).

2   Past life soul blocks and restrictions

Alice was told that she was an old soul due to the long length of her Akashic Records. The blocks and restrictions identified appeared during a lifetime in 17th-century Venice, suggesting that Alice had already completed a lifetime cycle and Alice was in a new cycle with a new life lesson to experience.

During the Venice lifetime, Alice was incarnated as a female, and was the eldest of five, having three brothers and one sister. Her father was a wealthy merchant who had good standing in the community and was very influential and innovative. He was involved in the selling and trading of silks and beautiful gems. Her father was a very difficult man, controlling, strong and judgemental. The value he put on his wife and daughters was much less than on his sons. When her father was out during the day the household was happy, but when he came home everyone had to be as quiet as church mice. If he went away on business trips a state of euphoria filled the home.

Around the time when Alice was 15 years old, one of her father's ships was lost which caused a disastrous crash in his business interests. He therefore arranged a marriage for Alice to save the family's honour and business. This created a pact (an agreement between her and her father) and the energy of this pact was around judgement, making Alice responsible for saving the family's reputation, business, and honour. Alice wanted to rebel but she wasn't allowed. The man Alice was forced to marry was similar in personality to her father and it was a very difficult relationship. He was a great businessman with a wonderful reputation, but underneath the surface he was a cruel man, a gambler and womaniser. The pact would continue to impact on Alice in subsequent lifetimes in that she would do whatever she could to repair situations even though she was not the root cause.

When her husband went away on business trips Alice became the power behind the throne. Although there was a male overseer, Alice was heavily involved in the running of the business and generating creative ideas, but this had to be kept hidden. Alice became quite close with the overseer and they possibly had a romantic relationship. Alice managed to create a wonderfully strong business, she forged trade and alliances in different places, but she was unable to get any credit for the work she did. This created a binding, which was about secrecy. Bindings occur when someone surrenders their free will to another person. Alice bound herself to secrecy for fear of being found out and this created a situation of being judged as being one person, but not getting credit for who she was, which was very debilitating. Whenever she interacted with her family she would receive criticism. She felt bound to be a passive person in order to protect her mother and sister. She was not in a position to get a divorce and the pact previously created with her father would have prevented this at a soul level.

When Alice married her husband she took two vows. The first was a vow of obedience to love, honour, and obey but she also vowed to obey her father. This vow continued to impact on all her relationships, perceiving that she has to obey others' orders, whether it is with family, work colleagues, friends, etc. Alice is likely to attract people into her life in situations where she automatically gives others the power, seeks approval from others, and often gets criticism in return. The second vow was a vow of chastity, where she refused in that lifetime to have children with her difficult husband. In subsequent lifetimes this vow could mean it is difficult to create especially where having children is concerned.

The secrecy that Alice had to maintain about her relationship with the overseer caused a lot of pain. The overseer felt ashamed for taking the praise for business success. The relationship was discovered 10 years later by her husband and the overseer was banished. Alice adopted the blame for this, which led to unjustified negative karma. This would continue to affect her in subsequent lifetimes, when she would give up her power to cover up other's wrong-doing and take the blame for their downfall, maintaining the belief that 'I should have done more.'

Alice received a great deal of judgement from her family and husband about being a bad person. Alice then had to face a life with a husband in charge who insisted that she continue with her great business ideas while he took the credit. Alice also had a soulmate contract with her father in that lifetime, he is possibly also her father in this lifetime. Soulmate contracts are not romantic, are often made with a close family member and can be quite toxic. In soulmate contracts, souls end up coming back to each other over and over again, repeating patterns, aiming to heal and teach each soul. Once this contract is cleared, it releases two people from the need to constantly repeat this pattern.

The Venice lifetime was very traumatic to Alice, causing damage to two of her chakras. A tear happened in both her heart chakra and throat chakra. The heart chakra is all about self-love and if she feels judged or criticised she is likely to struggle with self-love and her heart will feel weary. The throat chakra is about self-expression and covers the areas of the lung, throat, jaw, teeth, and ears and is all about communication. She may find herself to be good at talking but not feel that her voice is heard.

Alice also experienced some Godspark damage, which is the energy line from the Divine that provides a limitless supply of positive loving energy. When this is damaged, a person can lose faith in themselves and their spiritual faith. Alice's energy levels have been reduced due to this damage, which also makes her susceptible to sourcing energy from negative situations around her. Finally, Alice experienced some soul facet loss, which occurs when someone has experienced a significant trauma.

At the end of her session with Liz, Alice was given an opportunity to discuss what she had heard and whether she felt it related to current lifetime difficulties. Alice discussed the issues with her father in this lifetime and could see many parallels in the stories, especially around the relationship with her father when 15 years old. She could also relate to how the different blocks and restrictions impacted on her in this lifetime, including the vow of obedience and vow of chastity – having been told she may not conceive. Alice felt that she recognised the soulmate contract between her and her father which was about healing. She reflected on how she has been working at healing her relationship with her father during this lifetime despite the abuse she experienced as a child.

Summary of Alice

Alice was stunned by the similarities of her own past life story with her current life. What also convinced her of what she discovered from her Akashic Record work is that at the time of her reading she hadn't revealed to me her difficult relationship with her father. Alice therefore knew that I hadn't been speaking to my colleague. I hope that some of the similarities between my assessment and her Akashic Record reading are evident, in particular around her relationship with her father. The critical timings of the abuse with her father in this lifetime and the pact made with her father in her past life were identical – 15 years old. Her working careers in both lifetimes are similar, running successful creative businesses. In addition to the work with myself, soul level healing using the Akashic Records helped free Alice up to make new choices moving forward to live a heart and soul led authentic life.

Case study 4: Supervisee

During supervision, my supervisee discussed how she noticed how her spiritual insight had become more awakened during a session with one of her clients. This supervisee was already very open to and embracing of her spirituality in her personal life, but it had become dormant or hidden away in her clinical work. We discussed how this client was acting as a catalyst and providing an opportunity for my supervisee to honour her more authentic self and allow her spirituality to come through in sessions when appropriate. She then discussed a personal experience 18 years ago, which had profoundly affected her at the time, described below.

The 'knowing'

The phenomena occurred some 18 years ago following my second Reiki attunement and when my spiritual journey was very young and my third eye must have opened. I saw many images clearly inside my head, mostly just pleasant sensations, images like a lotus flower, Christ, Buddha, light, and colours, which I considered to have been stimulated by the beautiful spiritual environment. It was new to me and a very satisfying experience. One of the symbols I saw was like a round metal disc (I still don't know what it was) it looked like some kind of an Aztec mandala with lines on it.

I must add that I was very fortunate to have trained with and been attuned by Reiki masters who travelled the world studying with masters of the various lineages. My word for them has always been 'eminent.' They believed it was vital to keep their Reiki pure and were selective as to whom they trained as masters.

My Reiki teacher suggested we write down our experiences of the attunement. Sadly I do not have a copy now, but I wrote an account of my experiences and the letter was stamped ready to be posted to my Reiki teachers. For some reason, I picked up the letter and could not post it. That night I went to bed and a strange physical feeling slowly started to come over me, an altered state of consciousness, I hadn't a clue what was happening at the time. I had a buzzing in my ears and tightness in my chest and felt held by this energy. I was aware enough to be thinking, my God what on earth is happening? I 'saw' clearly in my head the metal disc I had seen during my attunement a day or so earlier. The image of the disc opened out into my consciousness inexplicably to me. I was transported right into the disc; I was in that disc on each and every single road and path all at the same time. I was told 'this is the Pattern of Life' – 'this is your life.'

I then experienced an utter, total, complete, 'knowing' of my whole life; I knew everything, absolutely everything about my life in an instant of time. I was there actually moving along inside these pathways on this very pattern of my life, living, breathing, seeing. I knew about and observed each step I had ever taken and each step I was going to take. I saw the roadblocks that I had and would arrive at in my life; where I had, I would turn around, change direction and continue on my way in life. I knew everything about my life. I was 'one' with and inside this living waking image. I was totally conscious and knew that something completely inconceivable was occurring.

Then, as if this wasn't incredible enough, the pathway opened out and a further expanded awareness sensation began. At first it felt as if it was inside my head; the energy was powerful but gentle, and my consciousness expanded, slowly and calmly into a vast expansion of boundless, limitless, and endless infinity. I 'knew' everything, absolutely everything 'that is, ever has been, ever was, time without end.' I was shown 'knowledge of all life,' everything. I knew everything about everything inside out, back to front, the whole lot. The more this 'awareness' expanded the more I knew past, present, future was all in one, 'all knowing,' 'all seeing,' 'all feeling'; ubiquitous and omnipresent. My GOD! My mortal conscious mind and left brain started thinking; what on earth am I going to do with all this infinite knowledge and information about everything – life and the universe? How can I live knowing all this? Will I ever be the same? And then as slowly as it came on it subsided and calmly and beautifully left me with a 'knowing' and an 'understanding.' Only fragments of the experience remained, only knowing that I was allowed to experience what 'knowing' really is but that it was impossible for me as a mortal to hold that knowledge and live on earth.

After tasting this knowledge, I did not share it with many others, only two other people. I knew nothing and no one would understand and they would think I was mad. I avoided it, as I did not understand it and it scared me. I felt honoured but confused. Even now, I have shared with very few.

Actually, it could more easily be explained nowadays, as films like *The Matrix*, which wasn't out at that time, portray the zooming in and out of different realities and more recently, the film *Lucy* showed a girl with incredible knowledge and powers in true sci-fi style, showing a mind expansion … but she blew up in the end!

This was not my first awakening; I experienced a series of awakenings, all of which changed my life and I knew I could never be the same again, not in a bad way.

As innately, I already knew I was being 'groomed' for something, those words resonated deeply and try as I might to resist it was impossible. This resulted in an endless search and I was faced with many real-life challenges and lessons. Now I am my textbook for my 'work.' I confess still to a lot of avoidance and fear, which had added further to my challenges.

All I know now is that I trust my instincts; the stronger the feeling the more I am compelled to take notice, even though it is not always in agreement with my very sensible left brain. My avoidance creates more challenges to get me on track again. Do I learn? Sometimes!

During this supervision session we discussed HLP and how opening up to additional spiritual possibilities would enable my supervisee to enhance her clinical work. Encouraging my supervisee to embrace her spirituality allowed her to resonate spiritually with her clients, so that she could share her guiding light and knowledge and start feeling more satisfied, fulfilled and authentic.

11

My journey

Trust in dreams, for in them is hidden the gate to eternity.

Kahlil Gibran

I have chosen to include my journey in this book because if I hadn't 'walked the walk' this book would never have materialised. I understand and accept that now. I also decided to keep this section until the end, so that readers can digest the book without prejudice, opinions, or judgements about my own experiences and see it in the true light and spirit in which it is being told. It is what it is, I am who I am. I have tried to keep this story as neutral and as sensitively written as possible. Some parts of my life have been omitted because it isn't necessary to mention particular relationships as my intention is not to cause conflict or hurt to those involved. My life and authentic truth have also changed since writing the first edition in 2018 and I believe this version is a much more authentic representation of who I am now. At the end I will give a summary of some of the information I have discovered about my soul level blocks and restrictions using the Akashic Records.

My journey so far

I grew up with a father who had underlying psychological difficulties – these were never formally diagnosed but were evident in his behaviour and ability to relate to others. I never really managed to get to the bottom of his difficulties. He had a tough start to life; his mother died from Tuberculosis when he was four years old, leaving behind his father to bring up three boys. Although my paternal grandfather remarried, he was a rather difficult person and this took its toll on his sons in one form or another.

I also had some challenging relationships as I grew up, but I didn't realise the impact this was having at the time, it was the norm, but it did shape my core beliefs about myself and the world. I strived hard to be accepted and loved. At a young age I didn't long for the materialistic aspects. I just craved that inner sense of peace and contentment but was unsure how to achieve this and was therefore constantly searching. I now recognise that my early life experiences taught me the gift and

DOI: 10.4324/9781003613749-15

value of compassion and loving kindness. My mother left my father when I was 13 years old. I suspect there were times during my childhood when teachers had concerns about my well-being, but no support ever materialised. Somehow, I kept going with a firm belief that there must be something better in life. I found it hard to settle in schools, never feeling that I fitted in with most of my peers and was probably just very confused, lonely, and depressed. In essence I was a lost soul! I believed in God and was brought up a Catholic and that faith gave me strength through the lonely and dark times.

When I joined Sixth Form College I met a wonderful person, Anu Dewan – she was fun, bubbly, and we connected straight away at a soul level. Sadly, after three months together, I watched her step out in front of a lorry to cross and join me on the other side of the road. The accident happened straight outside the small-town hospital and I managed to run for help. I travelled in the ambulance with her and her mother to a larger hospital where they operated, but her injuries were too significant and she died that night. It felt like my whole life stopped, I had just found someone who I dearly connected to at a soul level and this was taken away from me. One could be confused as to why I was so affected by the death of a person after three months of knowing them. All I can say is that I knew Anu at such a deep level and that for the time we were together we were inseparable. I remember opening my advent calendar in my bedroom the morning after Anu died and there was a picture of an angel. I didn't realise the significance that this would have on my life, but I knew that it meant something and was a message from her.

The next few years were tough having witnessed someone you dearly love die. I didn't realise at the time I was suffering from PTSD, but the strain of this came out in other ways. Unfortunately I didn't know how to access support and my well-being seemed to go un-noticed, despite losing weight and being very unhappy. I channelled my energy into college work and the ambition of going to university. Interestingly I had initially aspired to go to medical school with Anu but following her death I chose to walk a different path and one that eventually led me into Clinical Psychology. It was only when I started my EMDR training over 20 years later that I was truly able to process and heal from her death.

My spiritual awakening was gradual at first, alongside moving slowly toward a career in Clinical Psychology. After university, I went travelling and bumped into a man in a guest house in Malaysia and knew instantly we were going to get married. This was just an intuitive 'knowing' – I recognised him at a soul level. This was the first stage of my healing process. I entered a steady loving relationship and I began to learn that I too was loveable and valued – it took some effort to achieve and even though we divorced 21 years later, I will always be grateful to him for this healing.

For some time life seemed to be moving at a steady pace with the usual life challenges. I was determined to become a Clinical Psychologist, and this eventually paid off. My heart pulled me in the direction of working with children and families and I joined a CAMHS team where I stayed for 11 years. Within one and a half years, I had my first child, a daughter who had a wonderful spark, a strong, determined personality and she was very bright and energetic. My son was born two years later to complete our family and he brought a different, sensitive energy into the household. I recognised my children at a soul level from the first time I laid eyes on them, again just a 'knowing' of having been with them before.

Over the next 10 or so years, life was full of its many challenges, especially juggling family life with work and also parenting children who were many years later diagnosed as neurodiverse. Within a space of a few years, my father-in-law, a wonderful, caring, and gentle man died, following a prolonged degeneration in his health. His first son, my half-brother-in-law, died seven months later of cancer. The following year, on my son's fourth birthday, I received an answer phone message from my paternal aunt telling me that my estranged father had ended his life the day before. I hadn't seen my father for at least 10 years. I can still visualise sitting by the telephone in complete and utter shock replaying the message. I knew that I needed to take responsibility and ownership of sorting out my father's situation; I couldn't expect anyone else to do this even though I had not spoken to him for 10 years. I was living 200 miles away, but with the amazing help from my cousins and aunt I managed to organise his funeral and take over the administration of his estate, which took seven months in total. Confirmation to the extent of my father's difficulties during this process were very evident; he had been living in complete chaos, he was a hoarder and had lived a lonely and confusing life, yet there was a part of him that managed to appear to the outside world as relatively able. I never felt anger toward my father, as I understood his own upbringing had been very challenging for him. However, in my 20s, I had needed to impose loving protective boundaries on our relationship and cease contact. I had to learn through this experience that I wasn't my father, I was my own individual being and I had choices of how to live my life so I didn't repeat generational patterns. Sadly, he couldn't be helped; he didn't have any psychological awareness of his issues. Through my experiences with him, I learned the gift of being able to understand the systemic impact of mental health problems as well as the importance of empathy and reflection which were instrumental in my journey toward becoming a Clinical Psychologist.

My first major spiritual leap of faith: For many years, working in the NHS had been tough: increase in workload, administrative responsibilities, paperwork, and continual additional demands from one's job. There was less and less time available to see clients and work therapeutically because of the paperwork and bureaucracy. While I had been contemplating leaving for several years, I am a risk-averse individual and the prospect of working for myself and the associated financial insecurity daunted me and acted as a barrier (or so my ego would like to tell me!). I had gradually started working privately, which I enjoyed; feeling freer to offer more breadth to my clinical work, rather than operating within very restricted and imposed referral criteria. I could readily offer trauma and attachment work; at the time these were areas that were not being offered as a service in the NHS. I had opportunities to explore more spirituality within my private therapeutic work and interestingly, just being open to this gave access to clients who were also seeking something greater in their lives beyond the physical dimension. Eventually the universe decided to give me a big push that led me to hand in my notice in the NHS. I realised I just couldn't carry on juggling so many different balls and requirements and had to take stock of my situation. My spiritual interests were developing at the same time and I had to let go of the fear and trust in the process and the universe – I took that leap of faith, jumping off the cliff and hoping that I would land safely. The universe has never let me down and I have since run a successful Independent Clinical Psychology practice.

My second leap of faith came a couple of years later when I decided to separate from my husband after 21 years of being together and 18 years of marriage. An extremely tough decision; not only because children were involved, but also because my ex and I had not seriously fallen out with each other. To all intents and purposes we presented to the outside world as a strong unit. While there were various reasons behind this decision, one of the key explanations I can give is that I was aware that we were both changing and our spiritual paths and were drifting too far apart. In truth I felt like my soul was exhausted and dying. I couldn't ignore what my soul was trying to communicate to me anymore; that we would all be happier if we were not living together. This was a major decision for me, a huge leap of faith, not only letting go of a family unit, but also the perceived shame of being a divorcee, as well as the uncertainty about what lay ahead from a personal, financial, and work perspective. For over a year I had to experience letting go of virtually everything I knew at an ego level that made me feel secure: a marriage, home, some friendships and belongings. The only certainty I had during this time was my children, my spirituality, and faith. After nearly two years on this particular journey I found a wonderful home, nothing like I had initially envisaged, but it provided for all of my and my children's needs and was an absolute blessing in my life.

My spiritual healing

It is impossible to separate my personal and spiritual journey as they are so inter-related but there are a few key areas of my spiritual healing that are easier to write about separately from the information above. I have been told by some of my spiritual advisors that this is a Master lifetime for me and that I have chosen to heal my own generational challenges as well as clear karmic relationships.

My healing using the Akashic Records

I had no knowledge of the Akashic Records before 2016. I learned about these through a friend and embarking on this healing really connected me to the spiritual principles of this book. Over the next few years I did three specific clearings on myself and 11 joint overlays with other significant people in my life. I also did some soul level clearing for my children so that they have the best chance in life moving forward. All of these Akashic Record clearings have helped me to understand why I have had various issues or challenges with people in this lifetime.

I have been told during my Akashic Record healing that my primary life lesson has been FAITH in all relationships. This isn't about my spiritual faith, because that has always been very strong. Instead it has been about faith specifically in relationships and also in situations. This theme is something I was told that I have been working on for many lifetimes! I have also been told about some joint lessons with other individuals: including integrity, generosity, Divine love, power, self-love, loyalty, and happiness.

I believe that my Akashic Record healings have identified and cleared numerous blocks and restrictions at a soul level. I have been told about many lifetimes and the stories behind the blocks and restrictions which I could personally recognise as being connected to certain challenges I have been reliving in this lifetime from a physical, emotional, and spiritual perspective. Based on what I have been told, I have cleared numerous contracts, vows, negative unjustified karma, chakra tares, negative thought forms, hooks (from other souls), imprints, illusions, beliefs, genetic imprints, and so forth. Clearing in this way is quite similar to using EMDR to process traumas. Once the clearing has happened and I integrate the learning at a conscious level, I no longer feel distressed or affected by situations or relationships – they are what they are. I believe that clearing the distress has meant that certain relationships are now easier for me to manage and live. This has also given me the strength to make new choices rather than repeat similar patterns of behaviour.

I have also been told through this work that I possibly have at least three, if not more, negative karmic relationships in this lifetime where I am the recipient. I believe I know whom they are with now and it makes complete sense based on what I have experienced in these relationships during this lifetime. My initial reaction was to run away and shut these people out of my life completely. I now understand that in order to help those souls heal from the negative karma, it has to be worked through by offering unconditional love and forgiveness for past traumas while maintaining protective boundaries – it cannot be cleared in any other way. While the bearer of the negative karma may not change, I can change how I handle the relationship moving forward and that makes all the difference.

Conclusion

You may be pondering why I am telling you about my own journey and personal experiences. It certainly opens me up to being very vulnerable, judged, or ridiculed! Perhaps it is because I suspect it will give more credibility to the message I am trying to portray in this book, because I have learned through my own experiences how beneficial spirituality has been on my own healing, giving me such inner core strength, determination, compassion, empathy, and intuition.

I cannot emphasise enough that I see myself neither as a victim nor as special in any shape or form. I take full responsibility for agreeing at a soul level to participate in all my experiences in every lifetime and get to a place where I can recognise the gifts and lessons that I have learnt along the way. I didn't have this insight for a long time and it took a lot of courage and strength to understand the full story. I have felt anger, hurt, deep sadness and a victim, feeling punished, rejected, judged, betrayed, and much, much more. In essence, I am learning over time to be proud of who I am and be self-accepting and if I encounter other people's judgements and criticisms I am learning to recognise that it is their challenge and ego that needs addressing, rather than allowing myself to enter the victim role. I wouldn't say I was 'enlightened' or even fully 'awakened,' although the spiritual work I have undergone throughout this lifetime, especially in the past decade, has increased my awareness and my ability to be more aligned with the Divine Source so that I can live a more authentic life. I will always have areas of my life that need healing, as well as the joint and everyday life challenges that enable me to keep evolving and awakening.

In my work as a Clinical Psychologist, it is not uncommon for individuals to reflect at the end of their first session with me that they have never spoken to anyone before about what has happened to them in their lives. They have carried around with them not only traumas and difficulties, but also the sense of shame and the fear of being judged, rejected, or criticised for speaking the truth. I am no different from them, I have kept my life very private except for a few close friends. Fortunately, there is gradually becoming more and more acceptance that 'mental health' issues or psychological trauma can happen to most of us at some stage in our lives. It is therefore important that we as a population start feeling confident in speaking out the truth, being honest to ourselves and others and being willing and open to accept support in overcoming these difficulties.

Trying to remain attached to nothing and not focusing on the outcome means that I can be open to opportunities that come my way. As soon as I set a goal or target, I may miss something that could take me on a different path, a path that may be more fruitful and beneficial to me and my spiritual journey. This takes TRUST and the ability to completely SURRENDER and RELEASE expectations and desires. It has taken me a long time to reach this place of trusting my higher self and the universe to guide me to know which direction is for my better good and authentic self. I can only do this if I live my life through my heart and soul. I have to practise what I preach and mindfully, heartfully and soulfully embrace and breathe through any fear or discomfort that arises along the process. Otherwise, this book would never have been written!

I have a dream. That one day everyone will be given the opportunity to heal at the deepest level possible, whether it is from trauma or negative karma from this lifetime or past lifetimes. Where people can be healed of all blocks and restrictions at a heart and soul level so that they have the choice to fully align with their Divinity and reach their highest potential. Where unconditional love and kindness and compassion will cancel out the destruction and hate of life and make this a better lifetime for us all and for future generations to come.

In Divine Love

Alexandra x

Part 5

Resources

Resources

Exercise 6

Enriching and draining activities

Below is a simple table to help you to identify activities in your everyday life that are either enriching or draining at a heart and soul level. On the left-hand side, identify enriching activities that make you feel good or alive, make your heart and soul sing for joy, and make you feel self-compassionate or self-loving. These may not be activities you are currently involved in but would like to start doing. On the right-hand side, try to identify draining activities that you are currently involved with that make you feel exhausted, overwhelmed and depleted. If you can, try to be quite specific about each activity, so instead of just saying 'work' or 'children', can you identify whether there is anything in particular with that activity that is either enriching or draining?

For each activity, identify how often you are engaged with this using the scale below.

0 Rarely (once a month or less)
1 Infrequently (few times a month)
2 Sometimes (once a week)
3 Often (a few times a week)
4 Very often (daily)

Enriching/uplifting activity	Score (0 to 4)	Draining activity	Score (0 to 4)

Review what you have put in the table – what stands out to you? Is your life balanced between enriching and draining activities or have you filled your life with more enriching activities or draining activities?

If there are more draining activities than enriching activities, what needs to change to balance this out? How can you increase enriching activities so that you start to feel stronger and more joyful at a heart and soul level? Try to stay connected with your heart and soul as you do this exercise rather than slipping into your ego.

Exercise 7

Enriching and draining people

Below is a simple table to help you to identify people in your life that are either enriching or draining at a heart and soul level. On the left-hand side, identify people that make you feel good or alive, make your heart and soul sing for joy, are compassionate, nurturing or loving. On the right-hand side, try to identify people who are currently involved in your life that make you feel exhausted, overwhelmed or depleted. If you can, and if appropriate, can you be specific about what is either enriching or draining about that person?

For each person identify how often you have contact with them using the scale below.

0   Rarely (once a month or less)
1   Infrequently (few times a month)
2   Sometimes (once a week)
3   Often (a few times a week)
4   Very often (daily)

Enriching/uplifting people	Score (1 to 5)	Draining people	Score (1 to 5)

Review what you have put in the table – what stands out to you? Is your life balanced between enriching and draining people or have you filled your life with more enriching or draining people? If there are more draining than enriching people, what needs to change to balance this out? How can you increase being with enriching people so that you start to feel stronger and more joyful at a heart and soul level? Try to stay connected with your heart and soul as you do this exercise rather than slipping into your ego.

Exercise 8

Positive referencing beliefs

It is very easy to get caught up in negative thinking which spirals out of control and affects our emotions. One way to try and tackle this is to try and make a list of some positive self-referencing beliefs about yourself. Saying these regularly throughout the day, from the moment you wake up, can help to balance out negative thinking and with time can even cancel out the negative thoughts. Below are some examples of positive affirmations that you may find beneficial. If you are struggling to believe these, try and choose the ones that your friends or family would use to describe you.

I am a good person
I am kind
I am compassionate
I am caring
I have a good sense of humour
I am thoughtful
I am empathic
I do the best I can
I accept myself for who I am
I am loving
I am generous
I am considerate
I am passionate
I am enthusiastic
I am intelligent
I am hard-working
I am fun
I am honourable
I am forgiving
I am a good wife/husband/daughter/son/sister/brother, etc.
I do the best I can
I am generous
I am gentle

Exercise 9

Positive affirmations

One way to help you with a specific challenge is to construct a positive affirmation that you write down ten times in the evening and say out loud in the morning. Repeat for ten days or as long as required. If during this time another situation arises and you would feel it beneficial to change your positive affirmation then by all means do this. The key is to have a positive affirmation that fits the situation or challenge you are going through and helps to reinforce a positive outcome that you can manifest.

Remember, *what you think you manifest*! So if you think everything is going to fail and nothing good will happen in your life, then this is more likely to be the outcome. However, if you hold on to more positive affirmations then these are much more likely to transpire. Be realistic and not too specific when you write your affirmations. For example, if you write 'I am going to win the lottery' then this may not happen! If you can change this to 'all my financial and material needs are met,' then this is much more likely to be manifested.

Below are some positive affirmations that you may wish to use, but do try and be creative and write your own too or take aspects of different ones to create your own.

I am open and willing to receive Divine love and guidance.
I am open and willing to receive unconditional love into my life.
I am open, I am willing and I am ready to receive love into all areas of my life.
I am open, willing and ready to shine.
I deserve happiness and success in all areas of my life.
I deserve to live life with joy and happiness.
I trust in the Divine Source to protect me and keep me safe.
I trust that all my needs will be met.
I trust and have faith in the Divine Source.
I choose to live life as my authentic self.
I choose to be happy and at peace.
I choose to live a life free of pain and suffering.
I choose to let go of all expectations and to live my life in the present moment.
I choose to move forwards in my life to find freedom and peace of mind.
I choose to live life through my heart and soul.
I choose to release my ego and live life through my heart and soul.
I choose to take ownership of my life and all it has to offer.
I am grateful and thankful for everything in my life.
I embrace life's challenges and see these as opportunities to learn and grow into my authentic self.
I trust, belief, respect and have faith in myself.
I am safe, loved and protected.
I welcome in to my life all opportunities that will help me learn and grow so that I can become the best version of myself.

I release all in my life that no longer benefits me from a spiritual perspective.
I am in a happy and loving physical relationship.
I honour myself.
I have self-love, self-compassion, self-belief, self-acceptance, self-awareness.
I accept myself for who I am and welcome love and compassion in all areas of my life.
I joyously release the past, I am at peace and I can move forwards with ease and joy.
I surrender and release all my worries to the Divine.
I live life with ease and grace.
I am proud, confident, and have the courage to be me.
I am free and proud to be me.
I radiate love and compassion into all areas of my life.
I am ready, open and willing to accept my Divine gifts.
I joyously accept goodness into my life.
I am at peace with myself and my life.
I shine as a radiant being and live life with joy, peace, and happiness.
I manifest happiness, joy, and love into my life.
I surrender and release all fears of the future.
I forgive myself and others.
My heart is open and willing to receive Divine love.

Exercise 12

Re-writing your life story using HLP

Re-writing your life story is an opportunity for you to reflect back on your life so far. This provides a chance to discover what you are currently holding on to based on experiences you have had and people who have been involved in your life at these times. Then, using HLP, you have the opportunity to re-write and re-frame your life story using the concepts already learnt. These include:

- Identifying challenges and traumas, blocks and restrictions, and repeated patterns in your life.
- Life lessons.
- Reasons why you have had experiences or encounters with people to learn, teach, or heal.
- What are the gifts that you can now take away from these experiences?

Step 1

The first part of this process is to write down your life story as you can recall it. Some parts may be stories you have heard from other people for example what your mother, father, siblings or other significant people have told you about when you were born or very young. At some level you may have internalised these stories and connected with underlying thoughts or ideas about yourself or others. It is helpful to break your life story into sections. Probably the easiest way of managing this is to break it down into decades:

- **First decade**   0 to 10 years old.
  This would include stories about when you were born, nursery school or play-group, and primary school.

- **Second decade**   10 to 20 years old.
  This would include secondary school, college or university (if you went), or the start of a working career or family or travel, etc.

- **Third decade**   20 to 30 years old and so forth.

Continue this to the current time in your life without rushing the process. It may be easier to work at it in one go or over a period of time – there is no right or wrong way of doing this.

For each decade I would like you to first write down your understanding or recollection of what happened just as it comes to you now. Try not to intellectualise this process and if you can, write from your heart rather than from your ego. Be aware of key significant life events that may have happened during each of these decades. Try to include both positive experiences as well as challenges. Don't worry about missing anything out, what comes to you during this process is what you need to connect with now and you can always repeat this exercise at a later stage if you feel necessary.

For each significant experience try to identify:

- Who were the main characters in each significant event, for example, mother, father, grandparent, sibling, friend, teacher, neighbour, work colleague?
- What actually happened between you and the significant people or between the significant others (you may have been an observer of other people's interactions, arguments or difficulties)? Are there any generational repeated patterns happening in your family?
- How did this make you feel?
- What did this make you believe about yourself?

Try to become aware during this process of any repeated patterns or themes.

Step 2

Now I would like you to review your life story by becoming the observer for each significant experience or challenge and identify:

- What was this challenge trying to help you learn in terms of life lessons?
- What were each of the main characters trying to teach or heal in you?

- What were you trying to teach or heal in them?
- What is/are the gifts that you can take away from those significant events?

Step 3

This final step is to re-write your story from your heart (and soul), incorporating the information you have discovered during Step 2. Observe how this process can help you to start making new choices or decisions in life moving forwards based on:

- Previous repeated patterns.
- Your understanding of life lessons.
- The process of healing or teaching others or yourself.
- The gifts that you can learn to take away from these experiences.

How does this make you feel using HLP on your life story and does this change your understanding of the experiences you have had? Be aware of whether there are still significant blocks that are making these new choices difficult to make. What do you think these blocks are trying to teach you? What would you like to change moving forwards and what do you want to start believing about yourself now?

Exercise 13

Re-writing current life challenges using HLP

Re-writing your current life challenges is an opportunity for you to resolve issues more quickly by identifying what opportunities these challenges are trying to provide you with so that you can make new informed choices. Using HLP, you have the opportunity to re-write and re-frame these current challenges using the concepts already learnt, including identifying:

- Everyday life lessons as well as your main life lessons.
- Reasons why you have had experiences or encounters with people to learn, teach, or heal.
- What the gifts are that you can now take away from these experiences?

Step 1

The first part of this process is to write down the story or narrative of a current life challenge/s. There is no right or wrong way of doing this. For each challenge, write down your understanding of what has happened or is currently happening, just as it comes to you now. Try not to intellectualise this process and if you can, write from your heart (and soul) rather than from your ego. Don't worry about missing anything out, what comes to you during this process is what you need to connect with now and you can always repeat this exercise at a later stage if you feel necessary.

For each current life challenge try to identify:

- Who are the key significant people during this time, e.g. mother, father, grandparent, sibling, partner, friend, teacher, neighbour, work colleague?
- What is actually happening between you and the significant people or between the significant others (you may have been an observer of other people's interactions, arguments or difficulties)? Are there any generational repeated patterns happening in your family?
- How does this make you feel?
- What does this make you believe about yourself?

Step 2

Now I would like you to review this challenge by becoming the observer. For each challenge I want you to identify:

- Who are the main characters?
- What character are you playing?
- What is this challenge trying to help you to learn in terms of life lessons?
- What are each of the other characters trying to teach or heal in you?
- What are you trying to teach or heal in them?
- What is/are the gifts that you can take away from this challenge – in other words what is this opportunity being presented to you to help you move forwards?

Try to start becoming aware during this process of whether there are repeated themes, either of situations or encounters with other people.

Step 3

This final step is re-writing your story incorporating the information you have discovered during Step 2. Observe how this process can illustrate how you can start making new heart (and soul) led choices in life moving forwards based on:

- Previous repeated patterns.
- Your understanding of your main life lessons and everyday life lessons.
- The process of healing or teaching others or yourself.
- The gifts that you can learn to take away from these experiences.

How does this make you feel about using HLP on your current challenges? Be aware of whether there are still significant blocks that are making these new choices difficult to make. What do you think these blocks are trying to teach you? What would you like to shift moving forwards and what do you want to start believing about yourself now?

References

Abrams, H. (2008). Towards an understanding of mindful practices with children and adolescents in residential treatment. *Residential Treatment for Children & Youth, 24(1–2),* 93–109.

Aggs, C., & Bambling, M. (2010). Teaching mindfulness to psychotherapists in clinical practice: The mindful therapy programme. *Counselling and Psychotherapy Research, 10(4),* 278–286.

American Psychiatric Association (1994) *Diagnostic and Statistical Manual of Mental Disorders: DSM-IV.* Washington, DC: American Psychiatric Association.

Angold, A., Costello, E.J., Messer, S.C., Pickles, A., Winder, F., & Silver, D. (1995). The development of a short questionnaire for use in epidemiological studies of depression in children and adolescents. *International Journal of Methods in Psychiatric Research, 5,* 237–249.

Armour, J.A. (1991). Anatomy and function of the intrathoracic neurons regulating the mammalian heart. In I.H. Zucker & J.P. Gilmore (Eds.), *Reflex Control of the Circulation* (pp. 1–37). Boca Raton, FL: CRC Press.

Armour, J.A. (2008). Potential clinical relevance of the 'little brain' on the mammalian heart. *Experimental Physiology, 93(2):* 165–176.

Beck, C.J., & Smith, S.A. (1993). *Nothing Special: Living Zen.* New York, NY: HarperCollins.

Bernstein, E.M., & Putnam, F.W. (1986). Development, reliability, and validity of a dissociation scale. *Journal of Nervous and Mental Disease, 174,* 727–735.

Blevins, C.A., Weathers, F.W., Davis, M.T., Witte, T.K., & Domino, J.L. (2015). The posttraumatic stress disorder checklist for DSM-5 (PCL-5): Development and initial psychometric evaluation. *Journal of Traumatic Stress, 28(6),* 489–498.

Brown, K.W., & Ryan, R.M. (2003). The benefits of being present: Mindfulness and its role in psychological wellbeing. *Journal of Personality and Social Psychology, 84,* 822–848.

Braud, W., & Anderson, R. (1998). *Transpersonal Research Methods for the Social Sciences.* Thousand Oaks, CA: Sage.

Braud, W., & Anderson, R. (2002). *Integral Research Skills Study Guide.* Palo Alto, CA: Institute of Transpersonal Psychology.

Campbell, J. (2012). *The Hero with a Thousand Faces (The Collected Works of Joseph Campbell) (3rd ed.).* Novato, CA: New World Library.

Caplan, M. (2009). *Eyes Wide Open: Cultivating Discernment on the Spiritual Path.* Louisville, CO: Sounds True.

Childre, D., & McCraty, R. (2002). Psychological correlates of spiritual experience. *Biofeedback, 29(4),* 13–17.

Chopra, D. (1996). *The Seven Spiritual Laws of Success: A Practical Guide to the Fulfilment of your Dreams*. London, UK: Bantam.

Doyle, O. (2014). *Mindfulness Plain and Simple. A Practical Guide to Peace through* Mindfulness. London, UK: Orion.

Dent, A. (2025). *Using Spirituality in EMDR Therapy: The Heart Led Approach*. Abingdon: Routledge.

Dispenza, J. (2017). *Becoming Supernatural: How Common People Are Doing the Uncommon*. Carlsbad, CA: Hay House Inc.

Dobo, A.J. (2023). *The Hero's Journey: Integrating Jungian Psychology and EMDR Therapy*. Melbourne, FL: Soul Psych Publishers.

Dura-Vila, G. (2016). *Sadness, Depression, and the Dark Night of the Soul: Transcending the Medicalisation of Sadness*. London, UK & Philadelphia, PA: Jessica Kingsley.

Dyer, W.W. (2013). *Stop the Excuses!: How to Change Lifelong Thoughts*. Carlsbad, CA: Hay House.

Engel, G.L. (1977). The need for a new medical model: A challenge for biomedicine. *Science, 196(4286)*, 129–136.

Forgash, C., & Copeley, M. (2008) (Eds.) *Healing the Heart of Trauma and Dissociation with EMDR and Ego State Therapy*. New York, NY: Springer.

Grof, S., & Grof, C. (2010). *Holotropic Breathwork: A New Approach to self-Exploration and Therapy*. Albany, NY: SUNY Press.

Golding, K.S. (2008). *Nurturing Attachments: Supporting Children who are Fostered or Adopted*. London, UK & Philadelphia, PA: Jessica Kingsley.

Hacker Hughes, J. (2017). Towards a biopsychosocialspiritual approach to psychological distress. *Transpersonal Psychology Review, 19(1)*, 12–14.

Hayes, S.C., Strosahl, K.D., & Wilson, K.G. (2016). *Acceptance and Commitment Therapy, Second Edition: The Process and Practice of Mindful Change*. New York, NY: Guilford.

Howe, L. (2010). *How to Read the Akashic Records. Accessing the Archive of the Soul and its Journey*. Boulder, CO: Sounds True.

Hughes, D.A. (2007). *Attachment-Focused Family Therapy*. New York, NY: W.W. Norton.

Ingerman, S. (2014). *Walking in Light: The Everyday Empowerment of a Shamanic Life*. Boulder, CO: Sounds True.

Irving, J.A., Dobkin, P.L., & Park, J. (2009). Cultivating mindfulness in HCPs: A review of empirical studies of mindfulness-based stress reduction (MBSR). *Complementary Therapies in Clinical Practice, 15*, 61–66.

Ivtzan, I., & Lomas, T. (2016). *Mindfulness in Positive Psychology: The Science of Meditation and Wellbeing*. London, UK & New York, NY: Routledge.

Johari, H. (2000). *Chakras: Energy Centres of Transformation*. Rochester, VT: Destiny.

Jung, C.G. (1959a). *The Archetypes and the Collective Unconscious* (G. Adler & R.F.C. Hull, Eds. & Trans.). In *The Collected Works of C.G. Jung*, Vol. 9, Part I. Bollingen Series XX. Princeton, NJ: Princeton University Press.

Kabat-Zinn, J. (1982). An out-patient program in behavioral medicine for chronic pain patients based on the practice of mindfulness meditation: Theoretical considerations and preliminary results. *General Hospital Psychiatry, 4(1)*, 33–47.

Kabat-Zinn, J., Lipworth, L., Burncy, R. & Sellers, W. (1986). Four year follow-up of a meditation-based program for the self-regulation of chronic pain: Treatment outcomes and compliance. *The Clinical Journal of Pain, 2(3)*, 159.

Kabat-Zinn, J. (1994). *Wherever You Go, There You Are. Mindfulness Meditation in Everyday Life*. New York, NY: Hyperion.

King, D.E. (2000). *Faith, Spirituality and Medicine: Toward the Making of a Healing Practitioner*. Binghampton, NY: Haworth Pastoral.

Knipe, J. (2015). *EMDR Toolbox: Theory and Treatment of Complex PTSD and Dissociation*. New York, NY: Springer.

Kroenke, K., Spitzer, R.L., & Williams, J.B. (2001). The PHQ-9: Validity of a brief depression severity measure. *Journal of General Internal Medicine, 16*(*9*), 606–613.

Kroenke, K., Spitzer, R.L., Williams, J.B., & Lowe, B. (2010). The patient health questionnaire somatic, anxiety and depressive symptom scales: A systematic review. *General Hospital Psychiatry, 32*(*4*), 345–359.

Laszlo, E. (2007). *Science and the Akashic Field: An Integral Theory of Everything*. 2nd ed. Rochester, VT: Inner Traditions.

Laszlo, E. (2009). *The Akashic Experience: Science and the Cosmic Memory Field*. Rochester, VT: Inner Traditions.

Linehan, M.M. (1993). *Skills Training Manual for Treating Borderline Personality Disorder*. New York, NY & London, UK: Guilford.

Lovett, J. (2015). *Trauma-Attachment Tangle. Modifying EMDR to Help Children Resolve Trauma and Develop Loving Relationships*. New York, NY: Routledge.

McKee, D.D., & Chappel, J.N. (1992). Spirituality and medical practice. *Journal of Family Practice, 35*(*201*), 205–208.

Marich, J., & Dansiger, S. (2017). *EMDR Therapy and Mindfulness for Trauma-Focused Care*. New York, NY: Springer.

McClintock, C.H. (2015). Opening the heart: A spirituality of gratitude. *Spirituality in Clinical Practice, 2(1)*, 21–22.

McCraty, R. (2003). *Heart-Brain Neurodynamics: The Making of Emotions*. Boulder Creek, CA: Institute of HeartMath.

McCraty, R., Atkinson, M., Tomasino, D., & Tiller, W.A. (1998). The electricity of touch: Detection and measurement of cardiac energy exchange between two people. In K.H. Pribam (Ed.), *Brain and Values: Is Biological Science of Values Possible?* (pp. 259–379). Mahwah, NJ: Lawrence Erlbaum Associates.

Moore, T. (2011). *Dark Nights of the Soul: A Guide to Finding your Way through Life's Ordeals*. Chatham, UK: Piatkus. (Original work published 2004.)

Mother, The (1972). *Collective Works of the Mother*. Vol. *16* (p. 247). Pondicherry, Sri Lanka: Sri Aurobindo Ashram Trust.

Napoli, M., Krech, P., & Holley, L. (2005). Mindfulness training for elementary school students: The attention academy. *Journal of Applied School Psychology, 21*(*1*), 99–125.

Newton, M. (2011). *Journey of Souls: Case Studies of Life Between Lives*. Woodbury, MN: Llewellyn.

National Institute for Health and Care Excellence (NICE) (2022). *NICE Guideline, Depression in adults: Recognition and management*. https://www.nice.org.uk/guidance/ng222

O'Malley, A.G. (2018). *Sensorimotor-Focused EMDR: A New Paradigm for Psychotherapy and Peak Performance*. Oxford, UK & New York, NY: Routledge.

O'Malley, A.G. (2024). Quantum EMDR (QEMDR); A guide for EMDR therapists. *The Science of Psychotherapy, 12(1)*, 42–71.

Parnell, L. (1996). Eye movement desensitisation and reprocessing (EMDR) and spiritual unfolding. *Journal of Transpersonal Psychology, 28*(*2*), 129–153. Retrieved from www.atpweb.org/jtparchive/trps-28-96-02-129.pdf.

Parnell, L. (2008). *Tapping In: A Step-by-Step Guide to Activating your Healing Resources through Bilateral stimulation*. Boulder, CO: Sounds True.

Powell, A. (2018). *Conversations with the Soul: A Psychiatrist Reflects Essays on Life, Death and Beyond*. London, UK: Muswell Hill.

Read, T. (2019). *Walking Shadows: Archetype and Psyche in Crisis and Growth*. London: Aeon Books Ltd.

Schwartz, R. (2023). *Introduction to Internal Family Systems: A Revolutionary Therapy for Wholeness & Healing*. London: Vermilion.

Segal, Z.V., Williams, J.M.G., & Teasdale, J.D. (2002). *Mindfulness-Based Cognitive Therapy for Depression: A New Approach to Preventing Relapse*. New York, NY: Guilford.

Shapiro, F. (2018). *Eye Movement Desensitisation and Reprocessing (EMDR) Therapy Third Edition: Basic Principles, Protocols, and Procedures*. New York, NY: Guilford.

Shapiro, S., & Carlson, L. (2009). *The Art and Science of Mindfulness: Integrating Mindfulness into Psychology and the Helping Professions*. Washington, DC: American Psychological Association.

Shapiro, S., de Sousa, S., & Jazaieri, H. (2016). Mindfulness, Mental Health and Positive Psychology. In I. Ivtzan, & T. Lomas (Eds.), *Mindfulness in Positive Psychology* (pp. 108–125). Oxford, UK & New York, NY: Routledge.

Siegel, D. (2010). *The Mindful Therapist*. New York, NY: W.W. Norton.

Siegel, I.R. (2013). Therapist as a container for spiritual resonance and client transformation within transpersonal psychotherapy: An exploratory heuristic study. *Journal of Transpersonal Psychology*, *45(1)*, 49–74.

Siegel, I.R. (2017). *The Sacred Path of the Therapists: Modern Healing, Ancient Wisdom, and Client Transformation*. New York, NY & London, UK: W.W. Norton.

Siegel, I.R. (2018). EMDR as a transpersonal therapy: A trauma-focused approach to awakening consciousness. *Journal of EMDR Practice and Research*, *12(1)*, 24–43.

Siegel, I.R. (2019). Spontaneous awakening in transpersonal psychology. *The Journal of Transpersonal Psychology, 51(2)*, 198–224.

Sorrell, M. (2019). *The wonder of stillness: Meditation for children. A practical guide for parents and teachers*. Stillness Publishing.

Spitzer, R.L., Kroenke, K., Williams, J.B., & Lowe, B. (2006) A brief measure for assessing generalised anxiety disorder: The GAD-7. *Archives Internal Medicine*, *166(10)*, 1092–1097.

Sulmasy, D. P. (2002). A biopsychosocial-spiritual model for the care of patients at the end of life. *The Gerontologist*, *42*, Special Issue III, 24–33.

Taylor, S. (2017). *The Leap: The Psychology of Spiritual Awakening*. London, UK: Hay House.

Taylor, S., & Egeto-Szabo, K. (2017). Exploring awakening experiences in terms of their triggers, characteristics, duration and side-effects. *The Journal of Transpersonal Psychology, 49(1)*, 45–65.

Taylor, S. (2019). Spontaneous awakening experiences. Beyond religion and spiritual practice. *The Journal of Transpersonal Psychology, 44(1)*, 73–91.

The Happy Buddha (2011). *Happiness and How It Happens: Finding Contentment Through Mindfulness*. Brighton, UK: Leaping Hare.

The Happy Buddha (2015). *Mindfulness and Compassion: Embracing Life with Loving-Kindness*. Brighton, UK: Leaping Hare.

The Happy Buddha (2017). *A Mindful Life: Who's This In the Shower With Me? How to Get Out of Your Head and Start Living*. Scotts Valley, CA: CreateSpace Independent Publishing Platform.

Tinker, R.H., & Wilson, S.A. (1999). *Through the Eyes of a Child: EMDR with Children.* New York, NY: W.W. Norton.

Tolle, E. (2005). *The Power of Now: A Guide to Spiritual Enlightenment.* London, UK: Hodder Mobius.

Tomlinson, A. (2012). *Healing the Eternal Soul: Insights from Past Life and Spiritual Regression.* Online/self-published: From the Heart.

Van der Kolk, B. (2014). *The Body Keeps the Score: Brain, Mind, and Body in the Healing of Trauma.* New York, NY: Penguin.

Villoldo, A. (2005). *Mending the Past and Healing the Future with Soul Retrieval.* London, UK: Hay House.

Walsh, R., & Vaughan, F. (1993). On transpersonal definitions. *Journal of Transpersonal Psychology, 25(2),* 125–182.

Weiss, B., & Weiss, A. (2012). *Miracles Happen: The Transformational Healing Power of Past Life Memories.* London, UK: Hay House.

Weiss, D.S., & Marmar, C.R. (1996). The Impact of Event Scale – Revised. In J. Wilson & T.M. Keane (Eds.), *Assessing Psychological Trauma and PTSD* (pp. 399–411). New York, NY: Guilford.

White, R.A. (1994). *Exceptional Human Experience: Background Papers.* Dix Hills, NY: EHE Network.

Wilber, K. (2000). *Integral Psychology.* Boston, MA: Shambhala.

Williams, M., & Penman, D. (2011). *Mindfulness: A Practical Guide to Finding Peace in a Frantic World.* London: Piatkus.

The WHOQOL SRPB Group (2006). A cross-cultural study of spirituality, religion, and personal beliefs as components of quality of life. *Social Science and Medicine, 62(6),* 1486–1497.

World Health Organisation (2013). *Guidelines for the Management of Conditions Specifically Related to Stress.* Geneva, Switzerland: World Health Organisation.

Zenner, C., Herrnleben-Kurz, S., & Walach, H. (2014) Mindfulness-based interventions in schools – A systemic review and meta-analysis. *Frontiers in Psychology, 5,* 603.

Zoogman, S., Goldberg, S., Hoyt, W., Miller, L. (2014). Mindfulness interventions with youth: A meta-analysis. *Mindfulness, 6(2),* 1–13.

Websites

www.ddpnetwork.org

The official DDP website offering information about training, resources, conferences and the parenting approach.

www.dharma.org

A website offering information about insight meditation tradition and retreats.

www.drirenesiegel.com

Information about classes, workshops, retreats and online distance learning courses, integrating psychotherapy with shamanic healing.

www.emdrassociation.org.uk

The official UK & Ireland EMDR website offering information about training, resources, finding EMDR accredited practitioners and consultants, courses and conferences.

www.thefourwinds.com

Information on the world's renowned school of energy medicine, offering retreats, online training, resources etc.

www.franticworld.com

The website that accompanies Mark Williams & Danny Penmans book, with links to further meditations and books, upcoming talks, events and retreats. Also has a forum in which you can discuss experiences and share these with others.

www.gaiahouse.co.uk

Meditation retreat centre offering silent meditation retreats with a Buddhist tradition.

www.headspace.com

Online support on how to learn to meditate with resources for children and adults.

www.heartmath.com

For information on Heartmath technology, training, coaching, research etc.

www.heartledpsychotherapy.com

The official HLP website.

www.liz-king.co.uk

For information and support on Akashic Record work, soul retrieval, past life regression, psychic guidance and so much more.

www.mindfulnessunleashed.com

Information on Mindfulness retreats, courses, workshops and teacher training.

www.regressionacademy.com

Specialising in Past Life Regression Therapy, Regression Therapy, between lives spiritual regression and hypnosis training in Europe, Asia and the United States. Also offers soul evolution workshops.

YouTube meditation exercises

There are many guided meditation exercises and meditation music available on YouTube. These are just some examples to get you going, but also explore for yourself and find what works for you and your clients.

'Ah Meditation' with Wayne Dyer (https://youtu.be/a3pWHKc3evQ).
'I am that, I am' by Wayne Dyer (2018) (https://youtu.be/HiTtEQ_X2o8).
'OM Meditation' with Wayne Dyer – The evening OMM mediation for gratitude (https://youtu.be/65QOYK0zn_Y).
'Mindfulness Breathing' by Alexandra Dent (https://youtu.be/27nD6cMDG7A).
'The New Extended Light Stream' by Alexandra Dent (https://youtu.be/0w0cF-qxl2w).
'Heartful Meditation' by Alexandra Dent (https://youtu.be/8_R--gJP2Bw).
'Soulful Meditation' by Alexandra Dent (https://youtu.be/PPBMVp8cPzM).
'Mindfulness Meditation. Body Scan' by Mark Williams (https://youtu.be/CyKhfUdOEgs).
'Mindfulness Meditation. Breathing Anchor' by Mark Williams (https://youtu.be/fUeEnkjKyDs).

'Mindfulness Meditation. 3-minute Breathing Anchor' by Mark Williams (https://youtu.be/rOne1P0TKL8).

'Mindfulness Meditation. Befriending' by Mark Williams (https://youtu.be/pLt-E4YNVHU).

'Mindfulness Meditation. Exploring Difficulties' by Mark Williams (https://youtu.be/nlEFKxGNPHk).

Index

Note: **Bold** page numbers indicate tables; *italic* page numbers indicate figures.

For Product Safety Concerns and Information please contact our EU
representative GPSR@taylorandfrancis.com
Taylor & Francis Verlag GmbH, Kaufingerstraße 24, 80331 München, Germany